ISBN: 88-87434-13-1

Editrice DOGMA® S.r.l.
Via Cadorna Pal. 3B
17100 Savona - Italy
Finito di stampare nel dicembre 2003

EUROPEAN GLAUCOMA SOCIETY

TERMINOLOGY AND GUIDELINES

FOR

GLAUCOMA

IInd Edition

ACKNOWLEDGEMENT
This work was made possible by
unrestricted educational grants from the following sponsors
ALCON
ALLERGAN
CIBA VISION OPHTHALMICS – NOVARTIS
MERCK SHARP DOHME - CHIBRET
PFIZER - PHARMACIA & UPJOHN
THEA

CONTENTS

CHAPTER 3 - TREATMENT PRINCIPLES and OPTIONS

CHAPTER 4 - TREATMENT GUIDELINES

Foreword

These Definitions and Guidelines for Glaucoma have been produced by the European Glaucoma Society with the aim of both improving our understanding of the glaucomas and in providing a rational approach to their diagnosis and management. This work is intended to complement existing scientific literature and textbooks and to serve as an aid in dealing with glaucoma in a rapidly changing medical, scientific and socio-economic environment.
The project was edited by the EGS Guidelines Task Force and was reviewed and approved by the Executive Committee of the EGS.
We are grateful for the constructive criticism and novel ideas put forward by many colleagues who are experts in their field. A special vote of thanks is due to the financial support of the sponsors who made this production possible.

Roger A. Hitchings
President, EGS

Executive Committee

Roger Hitchings (*President*)
Clive Migdal (*Secretary*)
Alain Bechetoille
Eric Greve
Guenther Krieglstein
John Thygesen
Carlo E. Traverso

The Guidelines Task Force

Carlo E. Traverso (*Editor*)
Franz Grehn
Gabor Hollo
Yves Lachkar
Clive Migdal
John Thygesen

The European Glaucoma Society website is: WWW.EUGS.ORG

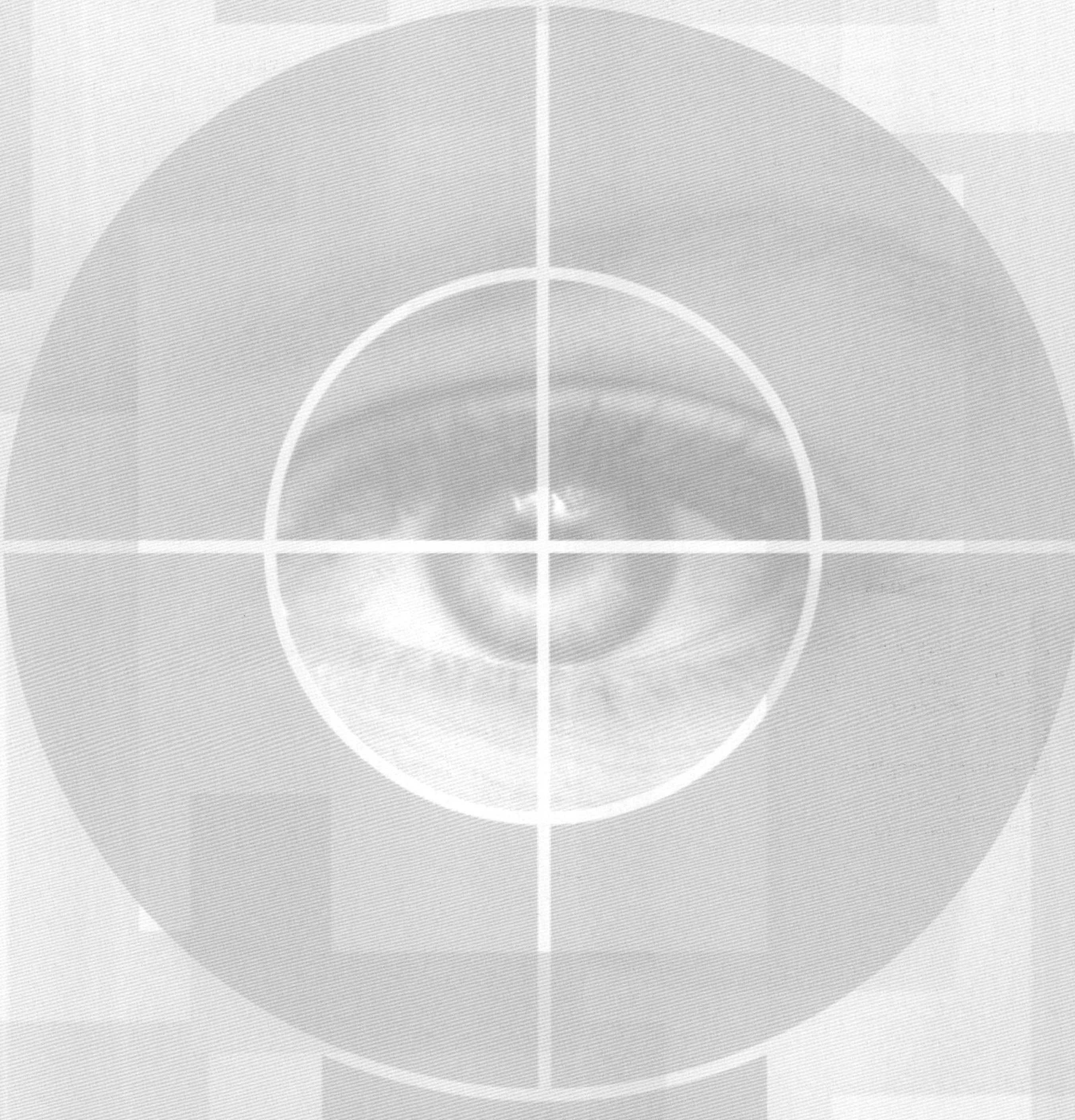

INTRODUCTION
CHAPTER

The aim of the book is to present in two main sections the view of the EGS on the management and diagnosis of glaucoma. The first part is devoted to the results of recent trials, flow charts, patient examination, terminology and classification. The second part is a reference section which tabulates available medical therapy, laser and surgical techniques. Our treatment guidelines are intended to support the general ophthalmologist in managing patients affected by or suspected of having glaucoma.The clinical guidelines are to be considered as recommendations. This work is based on glaucoma literature, conferences and clinical experience.
Our purpose is not to offer strict treatment protocols. Clinical care must be individualized to the patient, the treating ophthalmologist and the socioeconomic milieu. The availability of Randomized Controlled Trials (RCTs) makes it possible to apply scientific evidence to clinical recommendations.

The European Glaucoma Society (EGS), all contributors and sponsors disclaim responsibility and liability for any and all adverse medical or legal effects resulting directly or indirectly from the use of the guidelines.

I - TERMINOLOGY, CLASSIFICATION AND DEFINITIONS

Classification and disease definitions are arbitrary, and a consensus can be reached only if they are acceptable to most ophthalmologists on both theoretical and practical grounds.

The scope of terminology, classifications and definitions varies, however. As examples, prospective clinical trials, health planning, coding for third party payers, the review of existing clinical data and the classification of individuals for individualized treatment have somewhat different needs, and the level of detail and differentiation is not the same for all.
The following factors are to be considered in order to identify and separate the diagnostic groups.

1. *Anatomy* (see Ch. 1)

Open-angle, closed-angle, exfoliation, pigment dispersion etc.

2. *Function* (see Ch. 1)

Stage of ganglion cell damage, rate of decay etc.
Visual field examination, disc and nerve fiber layer assesment, rate of progression.
Techniques for imaging of the disc/RNFL are now available and still being developed and standardized (See ch. 1).

3. *IOP level* (see Ch. 1)

3.1 At which diagnosis is made (See Ch. 2)
3.2 At which damage occurred (See Ch. 1)
3.3 Target IOP (See Ch. 3.2)

Treatment principles
Once the type of disease is identified, the treatment goals appropriate for the specific individual are to be pursued.

A. *Treatment Goals* (See Ch. 3.1 and 3.2)

A.1. Quality of life
A.2. Quality of vision
A.3. Cost containment

In general, the goal of glaucoma treatment can be summarized as follows: preservation of visual function adequate to the individual needs with minimal or no side effects, for the expected lifetime of the patient, without any disruption of his/her normal activities, at a sustainable cost.

B. *Suggested ways to obtain the goal* (see Ch. 3 and 4)

B.1.	Selection of patients to be treated
B.1.1.	Identification of patients with disease
B.1.2.	Identification of patients at risk of developing the disease
B.1.3.	Treatment of the above when actual or expected rate of decay is likely to interfere with quality of life
B.2.	Decreasing the risk of ganglion cell loss
B.2.1.	Determine the target IOP for the individual In general, when there is more advanced damage, lower IOPs are needed to prevent decrease in quality of life
B.2.2.	IOP lowering
B.2.2.1.	Drugs Verify the short term effect on the stated endpoint in each individual i.e. IOP, blood flow etc. Confirm such effect in long term. When not effective, withdraw and substitute before adding a further drug Avoid combining drugs aimed at the same or similarly acting receptors Consider drug combinations which combine additive, different mechanism
B.2.2.2.	Surgery Compared with pharmacological treatment, surgery to achieves and maintains lower IOPs, with less diurnal variations, regardless of pre-treatment levels. Primary surgery, supported by large prospective studies, should be considered in selected individuals and/or specific environments
B.2.2.3.	Laser Verify the short term effect on the stated target IOP in each individual Confirm the above effect in long term When not effective, proceed to the next step to achieve the target IOP
B.2.2.4.	Verify the target IOP and the trends in the visual fields/disc.
B.2.3.	Enhancement of optic nerve blood flow (Ch. 1.5)
B.2.4.	Neuroprotection, neurorescue, neuroregeneration
B.3.	Incorporation of a quality of life measure in the outcome of treatment

C. *On-going quality control with independent evaluation of efficacy, safety, cost*

C.1.	Failures include patients suffering from the consequences of insufficient IOP lowering, unnecessary treatment, surgical complications, and progression of disease.

Since resources are limited worldwide, the following points are relevant to glaucoma treatment guidelines:

- support the prevention of visual disability in those at risk of decreased quality of life, avoiding widespread treatment of IOP per se;
- enforce effective IOP lowering in patients with large functional loss and/or rapid progression;
- implement population screening targeted at patients with unquestionable disease.

These points are supported by the results of Randomized Clinical Trials for glaucoma (See Chapter Introduction II).

It is important to stress that treatment guidelines are to be adapted to individual patients, socioeconomic environment, medical facilities, skills of the average ophthalmologist and of the health professionals, and resources available.

Rational and optimized care is not synonymous with automated therapy.

EVALUATION OF FUNCTIONAL LOSS/TIME FOR INDIVIDUALIZED TREATMENT

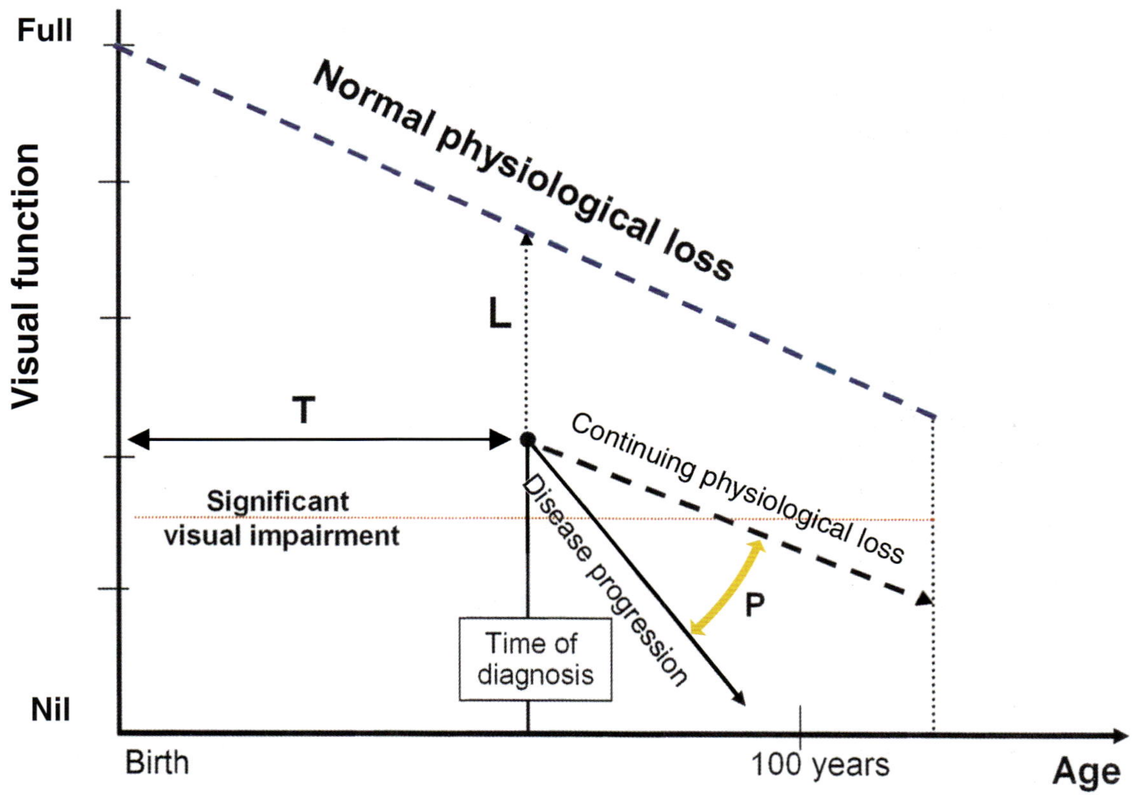

PRINCIPLE for ESTIMATING TARGET IOP = $\frac{\textbf{IOP}}{\textbf{L + P + Factors}}$

Fig. Introduction I.1
Evaluation of functional loss/time for individualized treatment
L = the difference of visual function between the normal for age and the function at the time of diagnosis
P = angle between physiological loss and disease progression representing progression rate
T = total functional loss at the time of diagnosis
FACTORS = individual features influencing clinical management (in alphabetical order)
1. Corneal thickness; 2. Family history; 3. Gonioscopy; 4. IOP range; 5. Life expectancy; 6. Pigment dispersion/PEX; 7. Stage of ON damage; 8. Stage of VF damage; 9. Systemic diseases

GLOSSARY

AION	=	Acute Ischemic Optic Neuropathy
ALT	=	Argon Laser Trabeculoplasty
BCVA	=	Best Corrected Visual Acuity
B.I.D.	=	Twice daily
CCT	=	Central Corneal Thickness
C/D o CDR	=	Cup-Disc ratio
Ch	=	Chapter
CPMP	=	Committee for Proprietary Medicinal Products (EMEA)
EMEA	=	the European Agency for the Evaluation of Medicinal Products
FC	=	Flow Chart
FDA	=	Food and Drug Administration (USA)
IOP	=	Intra Ocular Pressure
LTP	=	Laser Trabeculoplasty
MD	=	Mean Defect or Mean Deviation in visual field testing
MS	=	Mean Sensitivity in visual field testing
N.P.F.S.	=	Non Perforating Filtration Surgery
OH	=	Ocular hypertension
ONH	=	Optic Nerve Head
PAS	=	Peripheral Anterior Synechia
PEX	=	Pseudo Exfoliation
PSD	=	Pattern Standard Deviation in visual field testing
Q.D.	=	Once daily
Q.H.S.	=	Once daily at bedtime
Q.I.D.	=	Four times a day
QoL	=	Quality of Life
RCT	=	Randomized Controlled Trial
R/D o RDR	=	Rim-Disc ratio
RNFL	=	Retinal Nerve Fiber Layer
R.o.P.	=	Rate of Progression
Rx	=	Treatment
SWAP	=	Short Wavelength Automated Perimetry
T.I.D.	=	Three times a day
VA	=	Visual Acuity
VF	=	Visual Field

II - RANDOMIZED CONTROLLED TRIALS FOR GLAUCOMA

Since the first edition of the Guidelines the results from several large randomized controlled trials have been available. These trials addressed the effect of IOP lowering treatment in glaucoma have been published. Until these results, there was no scientific evidence that treament for glaucoma had any effect in decreasing visual loss from the disease. Many of the clinical recommendations given then are now reinforced by these results. Whilst a proportion of the recommendations and definitions in the second edition are still derived from common practice and consensus, it is now relevant to see how daily management of our patients can be helped by the findings of these studies. In the following pages we list each with a summary of their layout and results, outline strengths and weaknesses, and derive comments relevant to clinical decision making.

II.1 - THE OCULAR HYPERTENSION TREATMENT STUDY (OHTS)

Multicentre, prospective study on patients with a normal ocular examination, except for elevated IOP between 24 and 32 mmHg in one eye and between 21 and 32 mmHg in the other eye. The purpose was to study differences in conversion rate to POAG between the natural history (No Rx) versus treatment (IOP lowering Rx) in patients with elevated IOP (OH). To be eligible for recruitment, repeated VF and both clinical and stereophotography evaluations of the optic disc had to be assessed as normal by a reading center. VA had to be at least 20/40 in either eye. A total of 1636 patients between 40 to 80 years were recruited. Randomization was between treatment with IOP lowering medications and no treatment. The treatment goal was to lower the IOP to < 24mmHg and at least 20% from baseline, unless it was already <19mmHg. The majority of the patients were white non-Hispanic (1132) followed by African Americans (389), and a minority of other racial groups (87). The study design, the patient characteristics and the results are published in four different articles. Using 6-month visit intervals the minimum follow-up time was five years.
The primary outcome was the development of primary open-angle glaucoma defined as reproducible visual field abnormality or reproducible optic disc deterioration. All comparisons were made on an intent-to-treat base.

Summary of results[1]
The relationship between IOP lowering treatment and conversion to POAG was as follows: in the treated group the mean IOP reduction was 22.5% (SD 9.9), in the control group the decrease of IOP was 4.0% (SD 11.9). The cumulative proportion developing POAG at 60 months was 4.4% in treated eyes and 9% in controls ($p < 0.0001$): a 50% reduction of risk. The difference between treated and controls appears to increase with time. Self-declared African Americans recruited in this study showed larger cups and thinner corneas.
A large percentage of untreated patients (>90%) did not convert to POAG over time. Endpoints for POAG conversion were reached by both disc and VF findings in up to 10% of the cases, by disc only in around 50% and by VF only in roughly 40% of the total, without significant diferences between treated and control cases[2]. Among medication effects, 17% of those treated with a prostaglandin analogue showed iris or eyelash changes, versus 7.6% of those treated with other drugs ($p < 0.001$). Cataract formation was more in the medication group (6.4 vs 4.3 %; $p<0.06$). The incidence of POAG was higher than previously shown in epidemiological studies.

Baseline factors that predict the onset of POAG[3]
Baseline age, vertical and horizontal cup-to-disc ratio, PSD and IOP were good predictors for the conversion to POAG. The strongest association was with central corneal thickness (CCT); using a multivariate analysis on three groups composed of similar numbers but with decreasing CCT (> 588, between 588 and 555 and < than 555 micron respectively), those with thinner corneas had an hazard risk ratio of 3.9 compared to the thickest ones. The same higher risk for patients with thinner corneas was found when multivariate analysis was performed across the spectrum of IOP groups and cup-to-disc ratios.
According to these results, CCT-corrected tonometry readings are valuable when IOP measurements are high and treatment is being considered, since they will uncover falsely high readings caused by thick corneas[4].

- Strengths

Large sample size
Careful follow-up
Masked assessment of endpoints
Attribution of endpoints by a masked committee

Inclusion of all commercially available drugs
Careful quality control and feedback to technicians and photographers
True-incidence cases

-Weaknesses
Limited IOP range, i.e. no information on higher or lower IOPs than the selection criteria
Sample is from healthy volunteers and not population based
Relatively small number of POAG endpoints
Limited to patients with reliable visual fields
High thresholds for endpoints
Some risk factors under-represented
Criteria for conversion to POAG adjusted during study
If a correction factor was applied at baseline for CCT, up to 57% of white subjects and up to 37 % of black subjects would have corrected IOPs. If such an adjustment had been made at baseline some would not have had OH.
Some of the patients with normal white-on-white perimetry were later reported (ARVO 2002) to have had SWAP defects at baseline, thereby casting doubt on the "normal" state of some of the participants.

II.2 - COLLABORATIVE INITIAL GLAUCOMA TREATMENT STUDY (CIGTS)

Randomized clinical trial on 607 patients with newly diagnosed open-angle glaucoma
Initial treatment was either medication or trabeculectomy (with or without 5-fluorouracil)
A target IOP algorithm was used to guide the IOP lowering treatment.
Patients were treated as aggressively as needed in an effort to reduce IOP to a level at or below a predetermined target pressure specific for each individual eye
Primary outcome variables were VF loss and Quality of Life (QoL).
Secondary outcome variables were Visual Acuity (VA) IOP, Cataract formation.
Inclusion criteria were: (a) IOP 20 mmHg or higher with Humphrey visual field defect of at least three contiguous points and an optic disc which was considered compatible with glaucoma, or (b) IOP of 20 - 26 mmHg with two contiguous defect points in the visual field, or (c) an IOP of 27 mmHg and higher without visual field damage and suspected glaucomatous disc.

Summary of results[5]
On the basis of completed follow-up through 4 years and partially completed through 5 years, VF progression did not differ significantly by initial treatments.
IOP was lower with surgery (average 14-15 mmHg) than with medications (average 17-18 mmHg), decreasing 35% with medications and 48% with surgery. Perimetry results were equal and MD remained stabile in both groups. QoL was initailly better with drugs (mostly betablockers)
Both medications and surgery increased the incidence of cataract extraction (6% vs 17%).
Medical treatment (including cross-over) reduced IOP from 27 to 17 mmHg i.e. 10 mmHg or 37%. VA decreased initially more in the surgical group: it was equal at the end of follow-up.
ALT lowered the IOP after both medications and surgery.

- Strengths
Individualized target IOP approach
Newly diagnosed patients
QoL prospectively addressed

- Weaknesses
Inclusion criteria may have allowed recruitment of OH resulting in a case mix with little risk of showing progression
Sequence of treatment steps and cross over not clearly understandable
Initial trabeculectomy was sometimes supplemented with 5-FU
Follow up might not be long enough to show differences

II.3 - COLLABORATIVE NORMAL TENSION GLAUCOMA STUDY (CNTG study)

Multicentre prospective randomized trial comparing treatment versus no treatment in Normal Tension Glaucoma. The primary outcome measure was disease progression. To be considered for the study, patients had to have glaucomatous optic disc abnormalities and visual field defects according to standardized criteria[6], with no recorded IOP > 24 mmHg in either eye. After a 1 month wash out period and 10 baseline IOP readings (6 of them between 8 A.M and 6 P.M) the median IOP had to be 20 mmHg or less, with a maximum of one peak of up to 24 mm Hg. At least three reliable baseline visual fields (Octopus 32 or Humphrey 30-2) and at least 20/30 BCVA were required. Cases with far advanced damage, defined as less than 9 residual adjacent points measurable with stimulus size 3, were excluded. Ages ranged from 20 to 90 years.The follow up was every 3 months during the first year and and every 6 months thereafter. VF progression had to be verified on two or three fields performed within 1 month and confirmed in two or three fields done 3 months later[6]. Optic disc progression was confirmed by reading masked sets of stereo disk photographs.

Randomization. If the visual field defect threatened fixation or progression was documented i.e: recent VF progression, change in the optic nerve head appearance or disk haemorrhage patients were randomized to either IOP lowering treatment or as controls. A total of 140 eyes of 140 patients were randomized. Goal of the treament was a 30 % reduction from average of 3 baseline IOP readings, obtained with medications, excluding beta blockers and adrenergic agents, with laser trabeculoplasty or trabeculectomy, progressively stepped up to achieve the IOP goal. In patients undergoing surgery a 20% reduction was allowed without requiring repeated surgery.

Summary of results[7,8]

Treatment group: 61 eyes. At randomization the IOP was 16.1 +/- 2.3 mm Hg, during FU 10.6 +/- 2.7 mm Hg ($p<0.001$) . MD at randomization was -8.38 db (+/- 5.2)

Twenty eight eyes were treated medically or with Argon Laser Trabeculoplasty (ALT), 33 surgically.

A 30% IOP lowering was reached with medication and ALT 50% of the times.

Control group: 79 eyes. At randomization the IOP was 16.9 +/- 2.1 mmHg, during FU = 16+/- 2.1 mm Hg. MD at randomization was -7.54 db (+/- 4.3).

A 30% reduction from baseline was maintained in nearly 50% of the cases with medication, laser trabeculoplasty or both. Progression as defined by the protocol[6,7] occurred in 12% (7/61) of treated eyes and 35 % (28/79) of controls. No correlation with absolute IOP level maintained during follow up was found in either group. Kaplan-Meyer survival analysis showed that among those treated 20% progressed, 80% of the patients survived; among those not treated 60% progressed and 40% survived.

The 2:1 difference in *progression* between *untreated* and *treated* groups may be because progression was IOP related in a proportion of patients. Whether those who progressed in the untreated group would have been stable had they been treated is unknown.

Treated patients that progressed may be explained by their progression not being related to IOP or that their IOP was not at target. Cataract among treated eyes was 38% (23/61), with 48% (16/33) of those surgically treated and 25% (7/28) of those medically treated, and in controls 14% (11/79). A strong protective effect of IOP lowering was found only after the data were censored for the effect on VF of cataract formation[8]. The disease continued to progress in 20% of eyes even though the intraocular pressure had been substantially lowered (30% or more from baseline). Over half of those not treated showed no harmful visual field progression over 5 to 7 years of careful follow-up.

- <u>Strengths</u>

Long follow-up

Masked observers for VF and disc criteria

Three baseline VF required

Shows large IOP lowering effect from ALT and medications

- <u>Weaknesses</u>

Visual field criteria were changed during the course of the study[6]

No CCT values were taken at any time

IOP values up to 24mmHg are higher than usually defined for NPG

Patients with VF defects threatening fixation at baseline might not be progressive

Optic disc haemorrhage was used as a sign of progression for randomization into the study, but not as an outcome measure of progression

Far advanced cases were excluded

II.4 - THE ADVANCED GLAUCOMA INTERVENTION STUDY (AGIS)

Multicentre, prospective randomized study on advanced open-angle glaucoma patients who suffer from glaucoma that cannot be controlled by maximum tolerated medical therapy alone. The 591 patients of 35 to 80 years of age (789 eyes) were randomised between two treatment sequences for further interventions: argon laser trabeculoplasty → trabeculectomy → trabeculectomy (ATT) and trabeculectomy → argon laser trabeculoplasty → trabeculectomy (TAT). The second and third interventions were offered only after failure of the first and second interventions, respectively. The eyes enrolled had to be phakic, show a consistent elevation of intraocular pressure (IOP) of 18 mm Hg or greater, a reproducible, glaucoma-type visual field defect quantified using a custom made score system, as well as a minimum visual acuity equivalent with a Snellen value of >20/80. Patients with a MD worse than 16 db were excluded. Most of the patients were either Caucasian (325 eyes of 249 patients) or Afro-American (451 eyes of 332 patients). The study design, the patient characteristics and the results are so far published in nine different articles. Using 6-month visit intervals the follow-up time in these articles varies between 4 and 7 years.

Summary of results

Relationship between IOP and progression of the visual field damage over at least 6-years follow-up[9].

Predictive Analysis: eyes with average IOP greater than 17.5 mm Hg over the first three 6-months visits showed a significantly greater visual field deterioration compared to the eyes with IOP less than 14 mm Hg in the same time period. The amount of deterioration was greater at 7 years than at 2 years, i.e. increased with longer follow-up time.

Associative Analysis: eyes with IOP less than 18 mm Hg at 100% of the visits over 6 years did not show an increase of their initial visual field defect, whereas eyes that reached this value only at 75 to 100 %, 50 to 75 % or 0 to 50 % of the visits all showed a significant increase of the visual field defect. The amount of visual field decrease was greater at 7 years than at 2 years. These results indicate that *low IOP* and *low IOP fluctuation* are associated with reduced progression of a visual field defect in advanced glaucoma. Patients with the lowest range of IOP (max 18mmHg) were the only ones showing overall stability of average VF scores; this effect was well separated from the other groups only after the fifth year of follow-up. In this same group, 14.4 % of the patients showed worsening, and 18% an improvement of four of more units compared to baseline.

Relationship between treatment type and visual acuity /visual field preservation[10]: For a 7-year follow-up mean decrease of IOP was greater for eyes assigned to TAT, and the cumulative probability of failure of the first intervention was greater for eyes assigned to ATT. In Afro-American patients average percent of eyes with decreased visual acuity and visual field were less for the ATT sequence than for TAT. In Caucasians those were more favourable for ATT in the first 4 years, but then switched in favour of TAT. These results show that TAT sequence (trabeculectomy first) is recommended for Caucasians while ATT (laser trabeculoplasty first) is more favourable for the Afro-Americans. Adjustment for cataract progression[11] did not influence these results. Of course in clinical practice the choice must be individually adjusted to the patient characteristics and needs.

Risk of cataract formation after trabeculectomy[12]: The expected 5-year cumulative probability of cataract formation was significantly increased by the first trabeculectomy whether it was the first or the second intervention. Diabetes mellitus and higher age at the study entry were also risk factors. The of overall risk of cataract was 78 %. Complications of trabeculectomy (particularly marked inflammation and flat anterior chamber) increased this risk to 104% compared to uncomplicated first trabeculectomy (47%).

Racial difference in glaucoma progression after trabeculectomy[13]: Initial trabeculectomy retarded the progression of glaucoma more effectively in Caucasians than in Afro-Americans. Some patients continued to progress despite low IOPs; some patients retained high IOPs despite multiple interventions.

- <u>Strengths</u>

Long follow-up
Large sample
Standardized protocols
Elgibility measurements were separated from baseline measurements

- <u>Weaknesses</u>

The Predictive and Associative analyses were post-hoc
Only one visual field was used as baseline
Limited range of IOP during follow up

No stratification for stage of disease was attempted in the associative analysis
Patients with far advanced damage were excluded
Despite the title "Advanced Glaucoma" early cases of glaucoma were also included

II.5 - EARLY MANIFEST GLAUCOMA TREATMENT STUDY (EMGT)

Prospective randomized trial of treatment vs no treatment to evaluate the effectiveness of IOP reduction in early, previously untreated open-angle glaucoma. Secondary aims were to assess factors related to glaucoma progression, and to determine the natural history of the disease. During a population-based screening among 44,243 residents in Sweden, 316 eyes of 255 patients were recruited. Over 400 glaucomatous patients either refused enrollment or did not meet the entry criteria. 82.3% of patients with newly detected glaucoma had IOP values of 30 mmHg or less. All subjects were randomized to IOP lowering treatment vs no treatment. Treated patients had laser trabeculoplasty and received topical betaxolol twice daily in eligible eyes. Follow-up visits included computerized perimetry and tonometry every 3 months, fundus photography every 6 months. Decisions to change or begin treatment were made jointly with the patient when EMGT progression occured and also later if clinically needed[14].
Primary outcome measure was progression of disease, defined by sustained increases of visual field loss in three consecutive C30-2 Humphrey tests, as determined from computer-based analyses, or by optic disc changes, as determined from flicker chronoscopy and side-by-side comparisons of fundus photographs performed by masked, independent graders.

Summary of results[15,16]
A 25% decrease of IOP from baseline and a maximum absolute level of 25mmHg reduced the risk of progression by 50%. Treatment had positive effects in all groups of patients; with higher and lower IOP, older and younger patients, patients with early and later stage of disease.
Disease progression rates varied substantially between individual patients.
Risk of progression was less with a larger initial IOP drop induced by treatment.
The IOP level maintained throughout was related to initial IOP drop.

The mean Rate of Progression (RoP) measured as MD in dB/month observed for this study was:

	No Treatment	Treatment
dB/Month	0.05	0.03
dB/Year	0.6	0.36
dB/10 Years	6.0	3.60

Risk of progression decreased 10% with each mmHg IOP reduction from baseline to the first follow-up visit. Subjects randomized to the study had a mean baseline IOP of 20.6 mmHg and the IOP was < 25 mmHg in 80%.
Some patients did not show any disease progression even after several years without treatment. This study supports the idea that patients with lower risk for progression could be reasonably left untreated and followed closely as long as they remain unchanged, and that progression is related to disease stage.

- Strengths
Standardized protocol
Recruitment through a population-based screening
Strict crtiteria for examinations, independent observers.
Examinations carried out without expensive technology
Well designed assessment of VF progression.
Initial power calculations were based on the suspected difference in progression between the two groups.

- Weaknesses

Limited IOP range

Patients with advanced disease (≥16 Db) were excluded

Limited treatment options

High sensitivity of method for assessing progression may have reduced specificity

II. 6 - CLINICALLY USEFUL POINTS FROM THESE STUDIES

II. 6. 1 - from OHTS

1. 90% of OHT did not convert in 5 years, raising the 'need to treat' question.
2. Treatment is effective: of the approximately 10% that converted half could be prevented by the OHTS treatment. We do not know how much longer this treatment prevents further conversion.
3. It did not tell us what treatment would reduce the number of converters to close to zero.
4. The majority of conversion was based on ONH change: monitoring of the optic disc is essential for follow-up of OHT next to visual field. Will all disc changes eventually lead to significant visual field defects?
5. Conversion based on optic disc / RNFL changes (OHTS) may come before white/white VF changes.
6. Results on alternative methods for discovery of earlier visual function disturbances have not - yet - been published by OHTS. Preliminary SWAP analysis suggested that a proporton had VF defects at entry; this plus the suggestion of pre-existing disc change says that many already could have had POAG.
7. At a mean treated IOP level of 19.3 mmHg, 4.4% reached the endpoint. Delta IOP was 4.6 mmHg (<20%). Is this IOP reduction universally acceptable or just a pragmatic and achievable one?
8. Many persons with "Ocular Hypertension" measured by applanation tonometry do not have it because of thick corneas and should not be treated. Before the decision to treat is taken it is important to measure central corneal thickness (CCT) to evaluate the risk of conversion.
9. Not every patient with OH should be treated.
10. Offer treatment to OH patients at moderate to high risk taking into consideration age, medical status, life expectancy and likely treatment benefit.
11. Conversion to early POAG does not equal to reduced Quality of Vision (QoV).
12. Initiation of treatment is based on probability of decreased QoV, which is based on risk or on evidence of progression.
13. Risk evaluation can be guided by conversion rates from OHTS. Evidence is early damage and measured rate of progression. With a low risk profile no treatment is necessary (90% did not yet convert). Waiting for evidence of progression is reasonable as long as a good monitoring and call-back system is in place to avoid loss to follow-up. With a high risk profile treatment without waiting for evidence of progression seems acceptable.

II. 6. 2 - from CIGTS

1. Medical treatment (including cross-over) reduced IOP from 27 to between 17 to 18 mmHg or 37%. This level is often considered too high to prevent deterioration of the visual field in eyes with glaucomatous visual field defects.
2. The results show that medical treatment is able to reduce IOP considerably.
3. Inclusion criteria may have included a considerable percentage of ocular hypertensives resulting in a case mix with a reduced probability of progression. CIGTS does not contradict other studies due to the different case mix.
4. Surgical treatment reduced IOP from 27 to 14 mmHg i.e. 13 mmHg reduction or 40%.
5. Despite these differences in IOP, the visual field progression between the medical treatment versus the surgical treatment group was similar. This result may be explained by the complex and changing Target IOP determination approach used in CIGTS.
6. Study duration was too short and severity of disease too mild to be able to show a difference in medical versus surgical treatment.
7. The surgical group had more cataract extraction (17%, versus 6% in the medical treatment group). Medications may have produced cataract too, confirming the incidental findings of CNTG.
8. After 4 years there was no difference in visual acuity change between the two groups (including results of cataract extraction in the surgical group).
9. Quality of Vision questionnaires did not show important differences between the medical and surgical group.
10. At the start of the study 50% of patients worried about blindness, at the end 25%.

II. 6. 3 - from CNTG

1. Therapy that is effective in lowering IOP and free of adverse events would be expected to be beneficial in patients who are at risk of disease progression
2. The CNTG study shows that when IOP is lowered by 30 % the disease subsequently showed a lower incidence of visual field progression.
3. The protective effect of IOP lowering was found when the effect of cataract, largely caused by filtration surgery, was removed.
4. All results need to be interpreted considering that many patients in the untreated arm did not progress or progressed very slowly, many showed variable clinical course, with some progressing more rapidly.
5. Some of the treated eyes which progressed might have had IOP-independent disease, or the IOP reduction was not enough.
6. The study suggests that IOP plays a role in the progression of some of the NTG patients.
7. This was the first multicenter prospective randomized clinical trial to show that IOP reduction is effective in any type of chronic glaucoma.
8. This study concern patients with progressive NTG. 30% of NTG patients remained stable or for the duration of the study.
9. Trabeculectomy was used to achieve a 30 % decrease in IOP but was followed by cataract formation. In some cases this produced a decrease in visual acuity and an apparent worsening of visual field.
10. Drugs that are now commonly used were not available for this study. Results therefore overestimated the risk/benefit ratio that might occur in current ophthalmologic practice.
11. Maximum IOP values and/or pachymetry were not taken into account to try to determine which "normal tension glaucoma" patients will progress slowly and which will progress rapidly.

II. 6. 4 - from AGIS

1. IOP reduction reduces VF progression.
2. Different effects on progression at different IOP levels may not appear until 5 years or later.
3. A dose-response relationship between IOP and VF progression is likely.
4. Fluctuation may be an important aspect of the damaging effect of IOP.
5. Cataract formation is a side effect of glaucoma surgery, and it increases substantially with surgical complications
6. This was a post hoc analysis with residual doubt on results.
7. VF spread is very small; statistical significance achieved because of large numbers. A study that randomized for different IOP reductions is needed.
8. Whilst a dose relationship of IOP and VF progression is possible, is only one variable and thus may be difficult to unravel from other confounders.

II. 6. 5 - from EMGT

1. This is the first treatment versus no-treatment study of caucasian patients with early glaucoma and IOP ≤ 30 mmHg.
2. Limited but consequent treatment option (laser + betaxolol) of 25% IOP reduction moderately reduced progression from 62% to 45% (IOP from 20.6 mmHg to 15.5 mmHg).
3. Increase in lens opacity also occurred after betaxolol + laser and more than in the no-treatment group.
4. Progression may occur in half of patients having a 25% reduction of IOP.
5. Almost all progression was based on visual field data.
6. Side effects were acceptable.
7. Disc photos stereochronoscopy failed to detect visual field change. The disc changes were independently analysed.
8. The first Caucasian-only study to show that lens opacities follow medical/laser Rx.
9. Results may not be directly applicable to patients with glaucoma with very high IOP and with advanced disease
10. Results may provide information on the effectiveness of conventional treatment in most patients with glaucoma.
11. Patients should probably be followed more closely with visual function tests, during the first few years after being diagnosed, than commonly practiced.
12. Results do not imply that all glaucoma patients should receive maximum treatment.
13. Some patients do not show any disease progression even after several years without treatment. Mean progression

rate in untreated was 0-6 dB/year; many patients will never experience reduced QoL during their lifetime. Patients with lower risk of progression could be reasonably left untreated and followed closely as long as they remain unchanged.

14. Population screening for patients with undetected glaucoma shall be reconsidered, since in population studies in developed countries approximately 50% of all glaucoma patients are undiagnosed.

THE OVERALL PICTURE

These trials show that:

1. IOP reduction is of benefit in OHT/POAG of various stages. Unfortunately far advanced cases were not assessed
2. Lower IOP means better protection against visual loss
3. IOP lowering treatment will not inevitably be of benefit to all
4. Greater IOP reduction is not inevitably better for all
5. The vast majority of Ocular Hypertensives did not convert to glaucoma.
6. A 20% IOP reduction in OHT may not be sufficient to prevent conversion to glaucoma.
7. CCT measurements are unavoidable for the correct management of OHT.
8. CCT measurements have limited value for POAG assessment which is based on disk / RNFL and VF.
9. There is a large inter-individual variation in the IOP reduction / progression relationship.
10. Because of large interpretation variability of progression it may be reasonable to leave some (low risk) patients untreated and establish rate of progression first.
11. Large IOP reductions (40-50%) are needed in established glaucoma and even more so in advanced glaucoma if rate of progression threatens Quality of Vision.
12. All forms of treatment may increase the incidence of cataract, especially glaucoma surgery.
13. Side-effects of surgery expressed as Quality of Vision in the long run may not be widely dissimilar to those of medical treatment if cataract extraction is allowed as part of the treatment.
14. Disease progression increases with time.
15. A larger initial IOP lowering effect has a favorable influence on progression in later years.
16. Progression of glaucomatous defects does not necessarily mean a threat to Quality of Vision.
17. The aim of treatment need not to be no progression at all, but a reduction of rate of progression to such a level that Quality of Vision is not endangered during the patients lifetime.
18. It is important to differentiate between risk of progression, which may or may not require treatment vs evidence, that is confirmed worsening of VF/ONH, which may or may not require treatment, depending on the likelyhood of a decrease of Quality of Vision/Quality of life.
19. Patients of the OHTS and CIGTS where on average 10 years younger than those of AGIS and EGMT.

References

1) The Ocular Hypertension Treatment study. A randomized trial determines that topical ocular hypotensive medication delays or prevents the onset of POAG. Arch Ophthalmol 2002;120:701-703.
2) Feuer WJ, Parrish RK, Shiffman JC et al.The Ocular Hypertension Treatment Study: reproducibility of cup/disk ratios measurements over time at an optic disc reading center. Am J Ophthalmol 2002;133:19-28.
3) Gordon MO, Beiser JA, Brandt JD, , Heuer DK, Higginbotham E, Johnson C, Keltner J, Miller PJ, Parrish RK, Wilson RM, Kass MA, for the Ocular Hypertension Treatment Study. The Ocular Hypertension Treatment Study. Baseline factors that predict the onset of primary open-angle glaucoma. Arch Ophthalmol 2002;120:714-720.
4) Brandt JD, Beiser JA, Kass MA, Gordon MO, for the Ocular Hypertension Treatment Study (OHTS) Group. Central corneal thickness in the Ocular Hypertension Treatment Study (OHTS). Ophthalmology 2001;108:1779-1788.
5) Lichter PR, Musch DC, Gillespie BW, Guire KE, Janz NK, Wren PA, Mills RP and the CIGTS Study Group Interim Clinical Outcomes in the collaborative initial Glaucoma treatment Study comparing initial treatment randomized to medication or surgery. Ophthalmology 2001;108:1943-1953
6) Schultzer M. Errors in the diagnosis of visual field progression in normal-tension glaucoma. Ophthalmology 1994;101:1589-1594.
7) Comparison of glaucomatous progression between untreated patients with normal-tension glaucoma and patients with therapeutically reduced intraocular pressures. Collaborative normal tension glaucoma study group. Am J Ophthalmol 1998;126:487-497.
8) The effectiveness of intraocular pressure reduction in the treatment of normal tension glaucoma. Collaborative normal tension glaucoma study group. Am J Ophthalmol 1998;126:498-505.
9) The AGIS Investigators: The Advanced Glaucoma Intervention Study (AGIS): 7. The relationship between control of intraocular pressure and visual field deterioration. Am J Ophthalmol 2000;130:429-440.
10) The AGIS Investigators: The Advanced Glaucoma Intervention Study (AGIS): 4. Comparison of treatment outcomes within race. Ophthalmology 1998;105:1146-1164.
11) The AGIS Investigators: The Advanced Glaucoma Intervention Study, 6: Effect of cataract on visual field and visual acuity. Arch Ophthalmol 2000;118:1639-1652.
12) The AGIS Investigators: The Advanced Glaucoma Intervention Study, 8: Risk of cataract formation after trabeculectomy. Arch Ophthalmol 2001;119:1771-1780.
13) The AGIS Investigators: The Advanced Glaucoma Intervention Study (AGIS): 9. Comparison of glaucoma outcomes in black and white patients within the treatment groups. Am J Ophthalmol 2001;132:311-320.
14) Leske MC, Heijl A, Hyman L, Bengtsson B. Early Manifest Glaucoma Trial: design and baseline data. Ophthalmology 1999;106:2144-2153.
15) Heijl A, Leske MC, Bengtsson B, Hyman L, Hussein M, for the Early Manifest Glaucoma Trial Group. Reduction of Intraocular Pressure and Glaucoma Progression. Results From the Early Manifest Glaucoma Trial. Arch Ophthalmol 2002;120:1268-1279.
16) Leske MC, Heijl A, Hussein M, Bengtsson B, Hyman L, Konaroff E, for the Early Manifest Glaucoma Trial Group. Factors for Glaucoma Progression and the effect of treatment. The Early Manifest Glaucoma Trial. Arch Ophthalmol 2003;121:48-56.

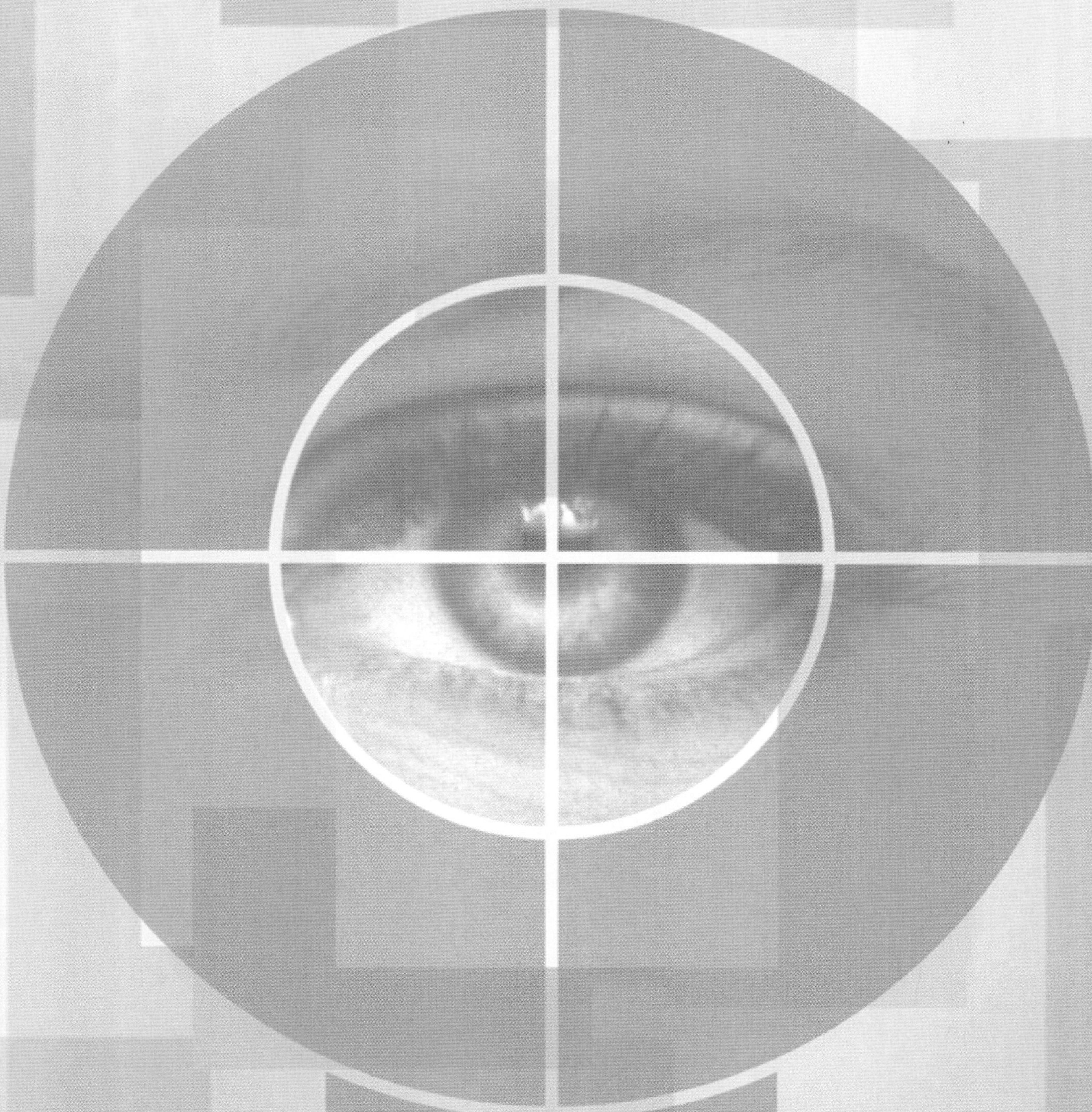

FLOW CHARTS

I - QUESTIONS TO ASK TO YOUR GLAUCOMA PATIENT

- How are you?

- How do you think your eyes are doing?

- Do you understand your diagnosis?

- Do you have difficulty with your daily tasks?

- Are the glaucoma medications interfering with your daily activities?

- Are you worried about your eyes?

- Do you think your condition is better, stable or worse?

II - DIAGNOSTIC CRITERIA

Primary Open-Angle Glaucoma and related conditions

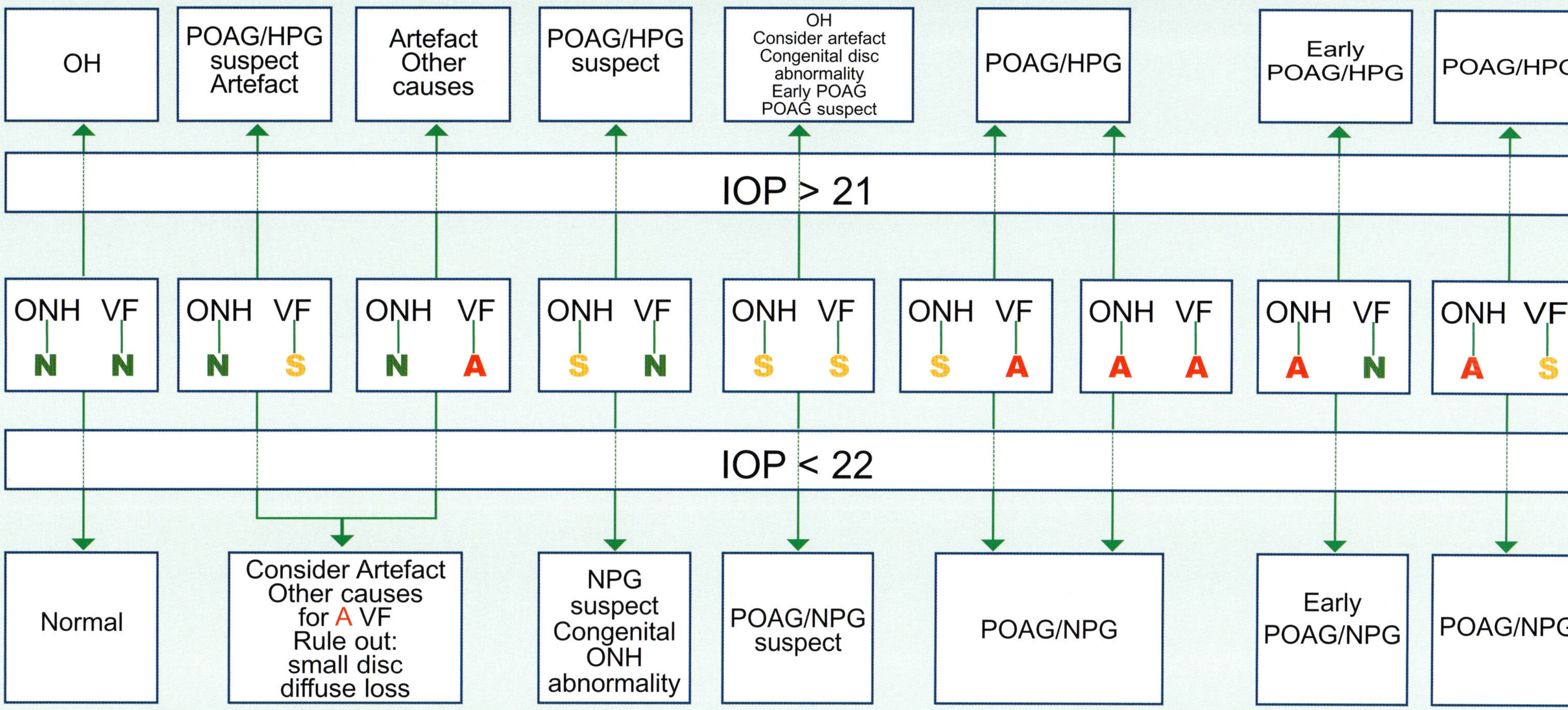

please see Ch 2.2
POAG has been arbitrary subdivided into High Pressure and Normal Pressure diseases, even though they may represent a spectrum of optic neuropathies variably sensitive to the IOP.

IN CASE OF FINDINGS THAT DO NOT MATCH, ALWAYS CONSIDER OTHER DISEASES AND ARTEFACTS

LEGEND

- OH = Ocular Hypertension
- POAG = Primary Open-Angle Glaucoma
- HPG = High Pressure Glaucoma
- NPG = Normal Pressure Glaucoma
- ONH = Optic Nerve Head
- VF = Visual Field
- N = Normal
- A = Abnormal
- S = Suspicious

III - ABNORMAL THRESHOLD VISUAL FIELD

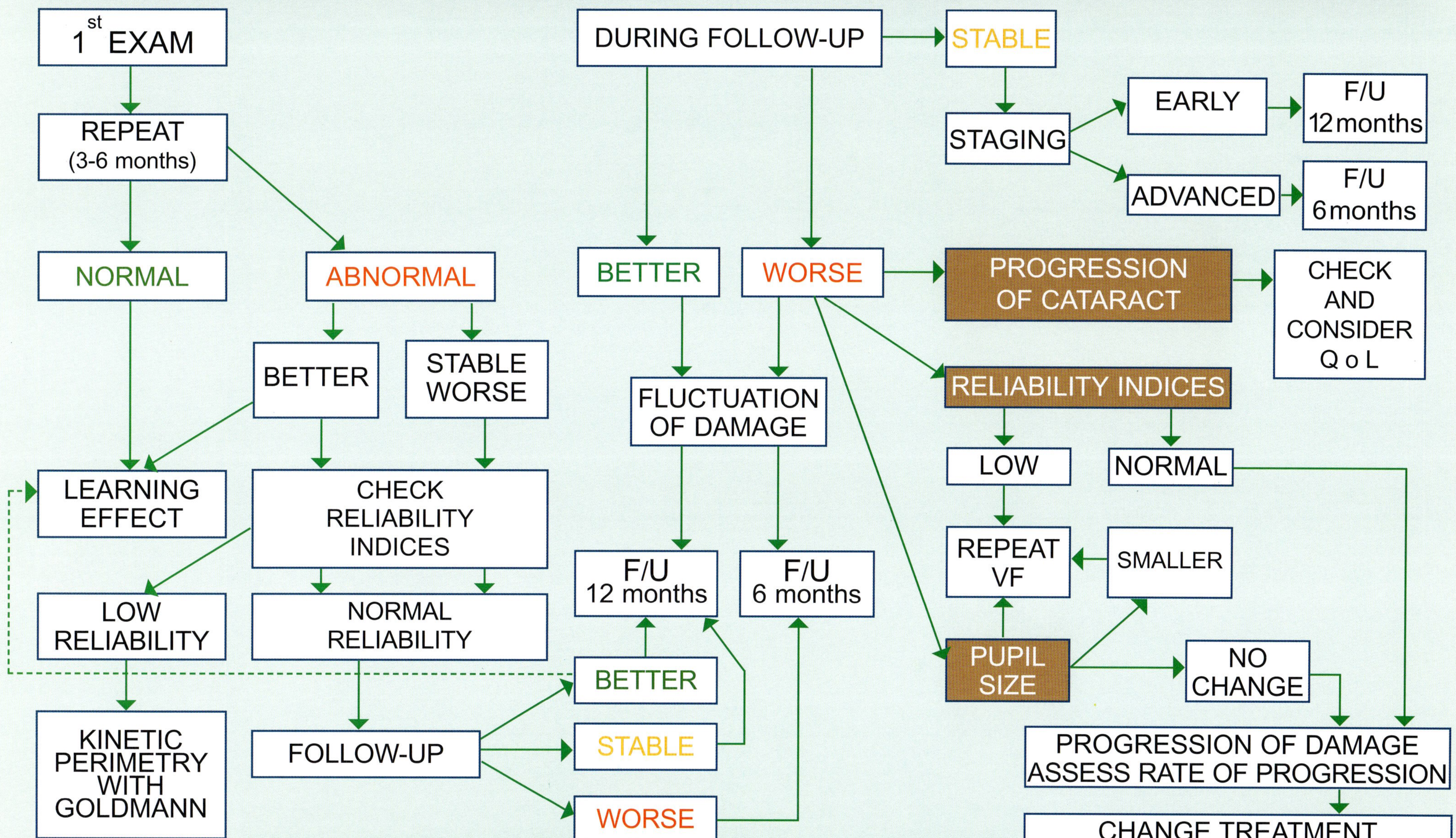

Before accepting VF defects as real, they must be cofirmed on two consecutive exams (excluding the initial one). Follow-up intervals are just suggestions.

IV - ASSESSMENT AND FOLLOW-UP

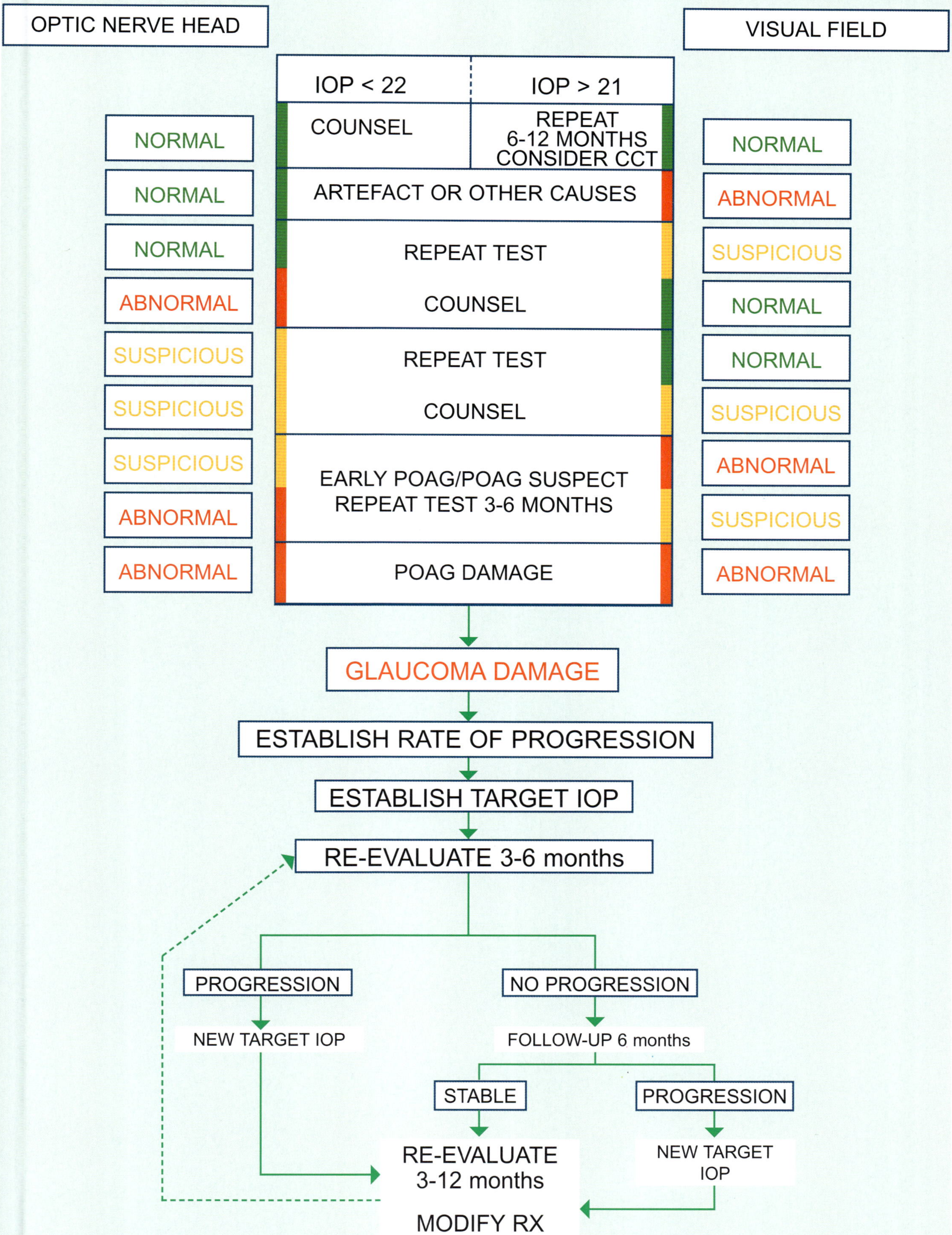

FOLLOW-UP INTERVALS ARE JUST RECOMMENDATIONS

V - GONIOSCOPIC OPEN ANGLES

SOME DIAGNOSTIC CLUES

POAGs	Normal Angle
CONGENITAL GALUCOMA INFANTILE GLAUCOMA	Angle poorly differentiated Trabeculodysgenesis (Barkan's membrane) Anterior insertion of the iris Posterior embryotoxon
PSEUDOEXFOLIATION GLAUCOMA	Black pigmented undulating line on or anterior to Schwalbe's line (Sampaolesi's line) Heavily pigmented trabeculum
PIGMENTARY GLAUCOMA	Mid trabecular band of brown pigment Pigment on Schwalbe's line
OPEN ANGLE GLAUCOMA SECONDARY TO UVEITIS	Scattered pigment, new vessels, peripheral anterior synechia
POST-TRAUMATIC GLAUCOMA	Angle recession, irregular iris insertion Possible increase of pigment
OPEN ANGLE GLAUCOMA SECONDARY TO NEOVASCULARIZATION	Neovascular membrane

VI - TARGET IOP

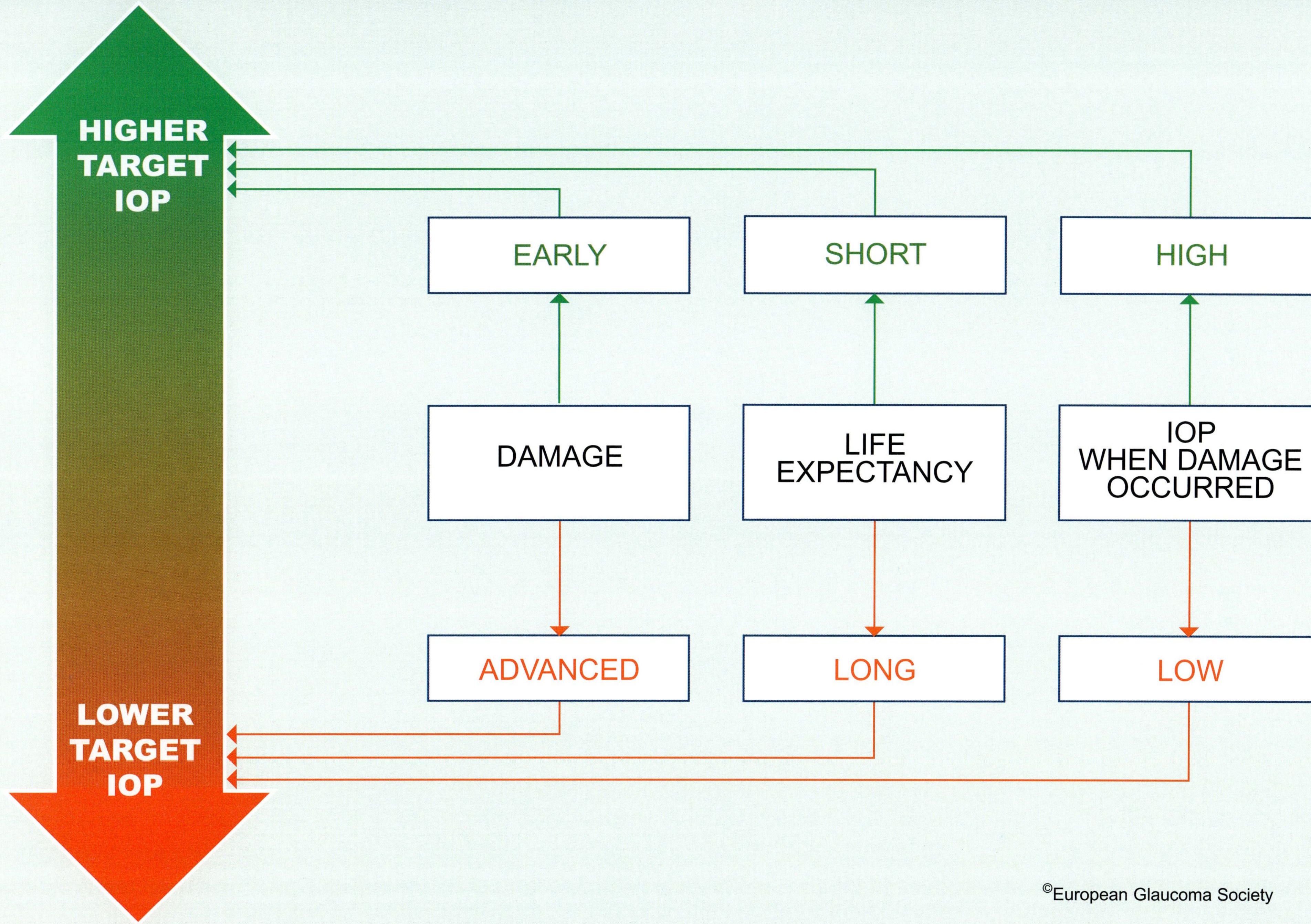

VII - TREATMENT STEPLADDER

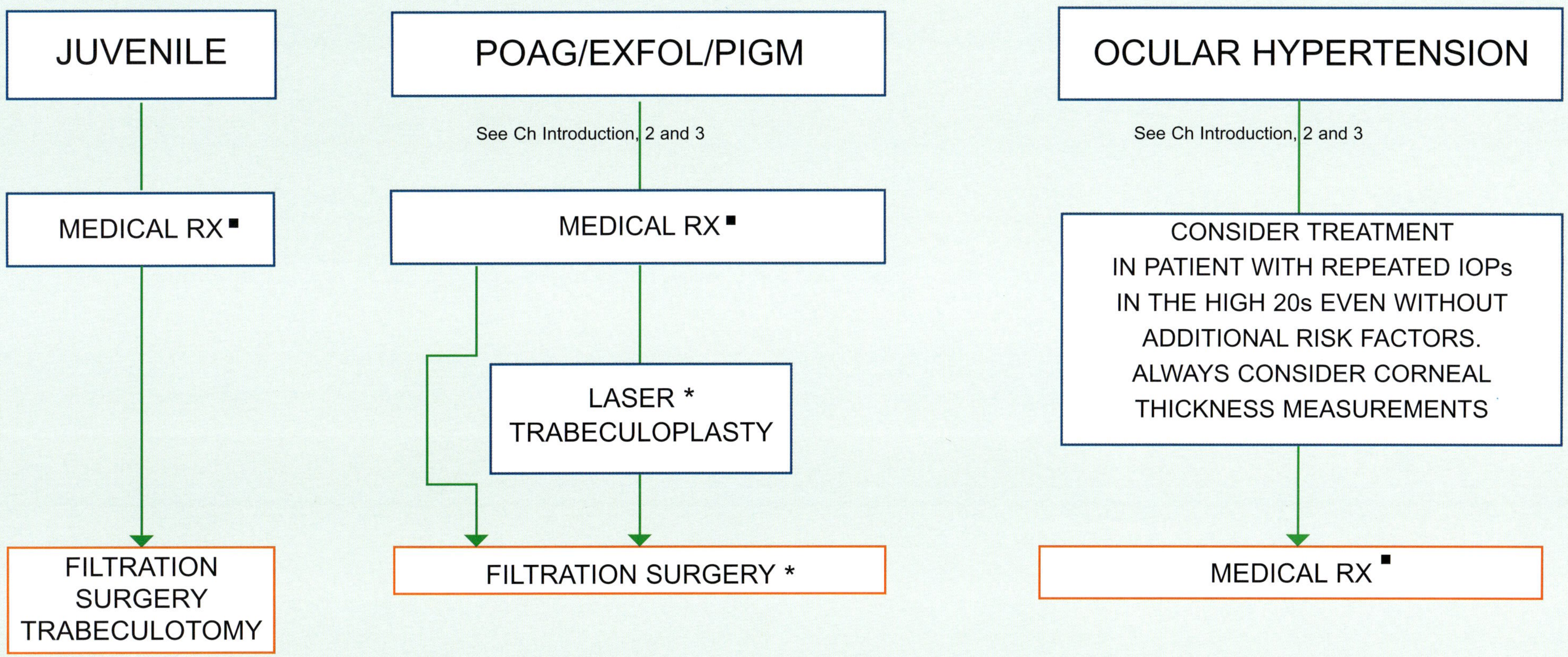

IF THE ABOVE NOT SUCCESSFUL, CONSIDER REPEAT FILTRATION SURGERY+ANTIMETABOLITES OR AQUEOUS DRAINAGE IMPLANCT OR CYCLO DESTRUCTIVE PROCEDURE

* In certains cases, it may be necessary to consider filtration surgery without resorting to laser trabeculoplasty

■ up to 2-3 different drugs. Do not add a drug to a non-effective one; consider switching

VIII - THERAPEUTIC TRIAL OF GLAUCOMA MEDICATIONS

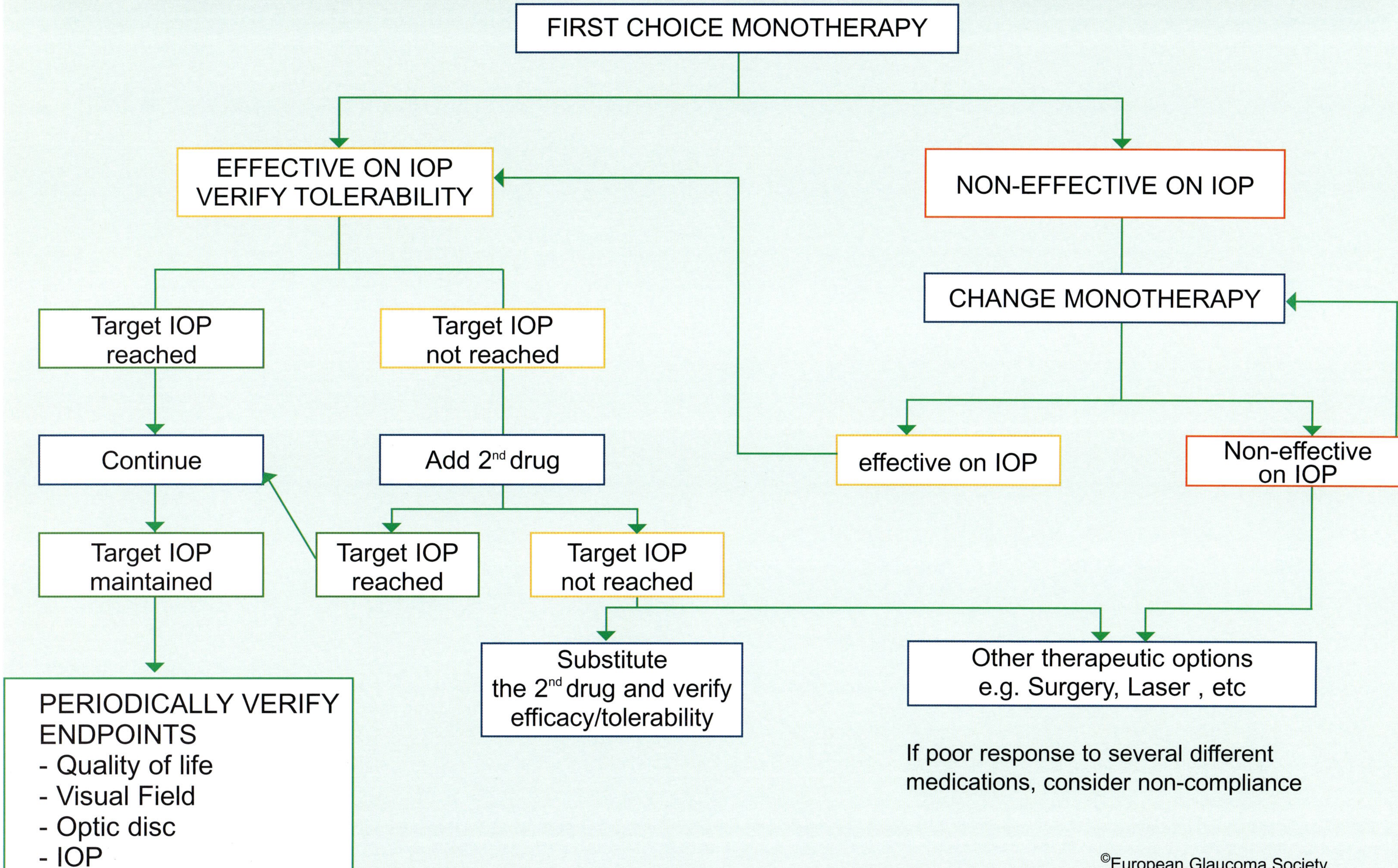

IX - MONOTHERAPY

(in alphabetic order)

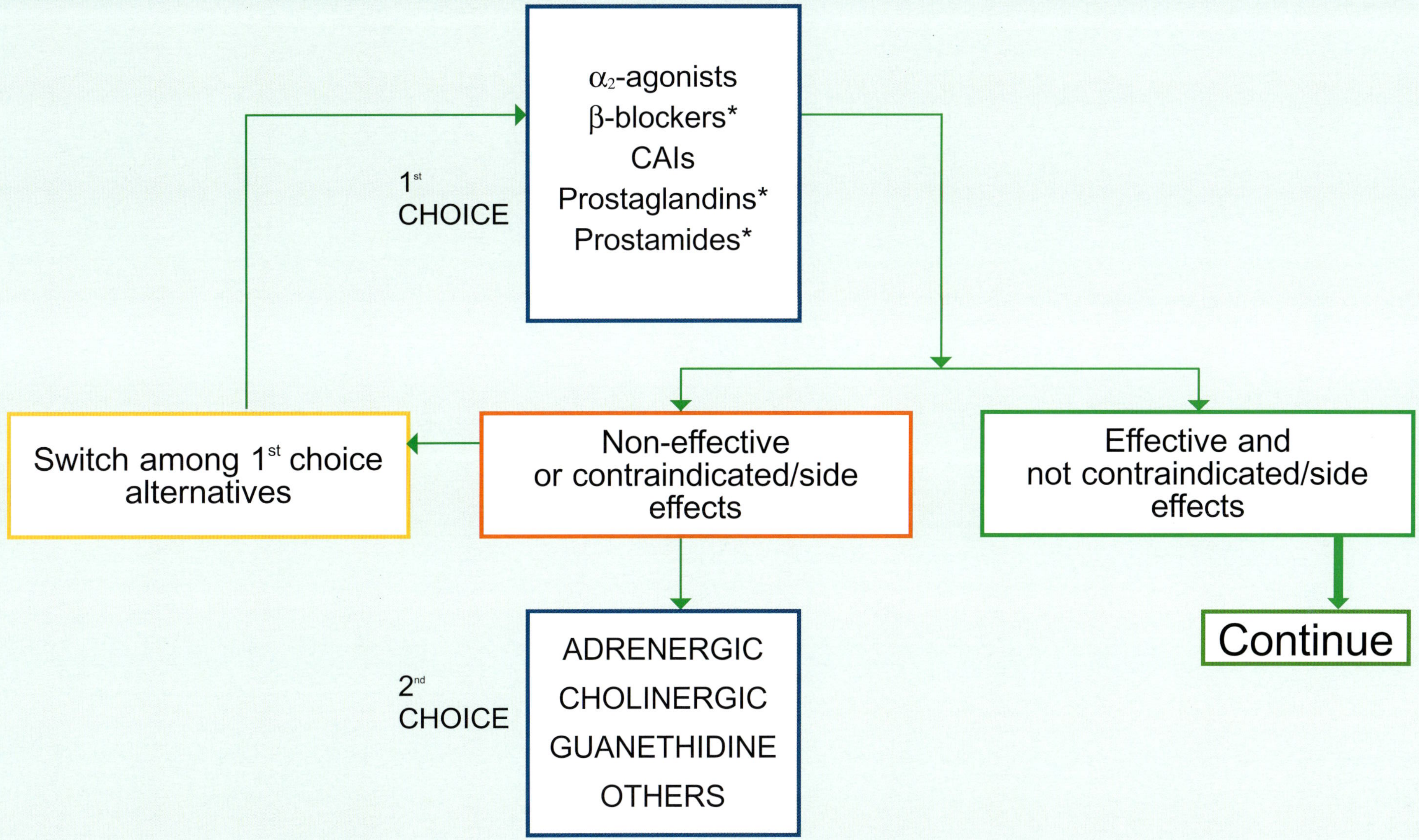

*β-blockers, latanoprost and travoprost are approved by regulatory bodies as first-line treatment; an application has also been made for bimatoprost

see also ch. 3.3, flow chart VIII

X - CAUSAL APPROACH TO ANGLE CLOSURE

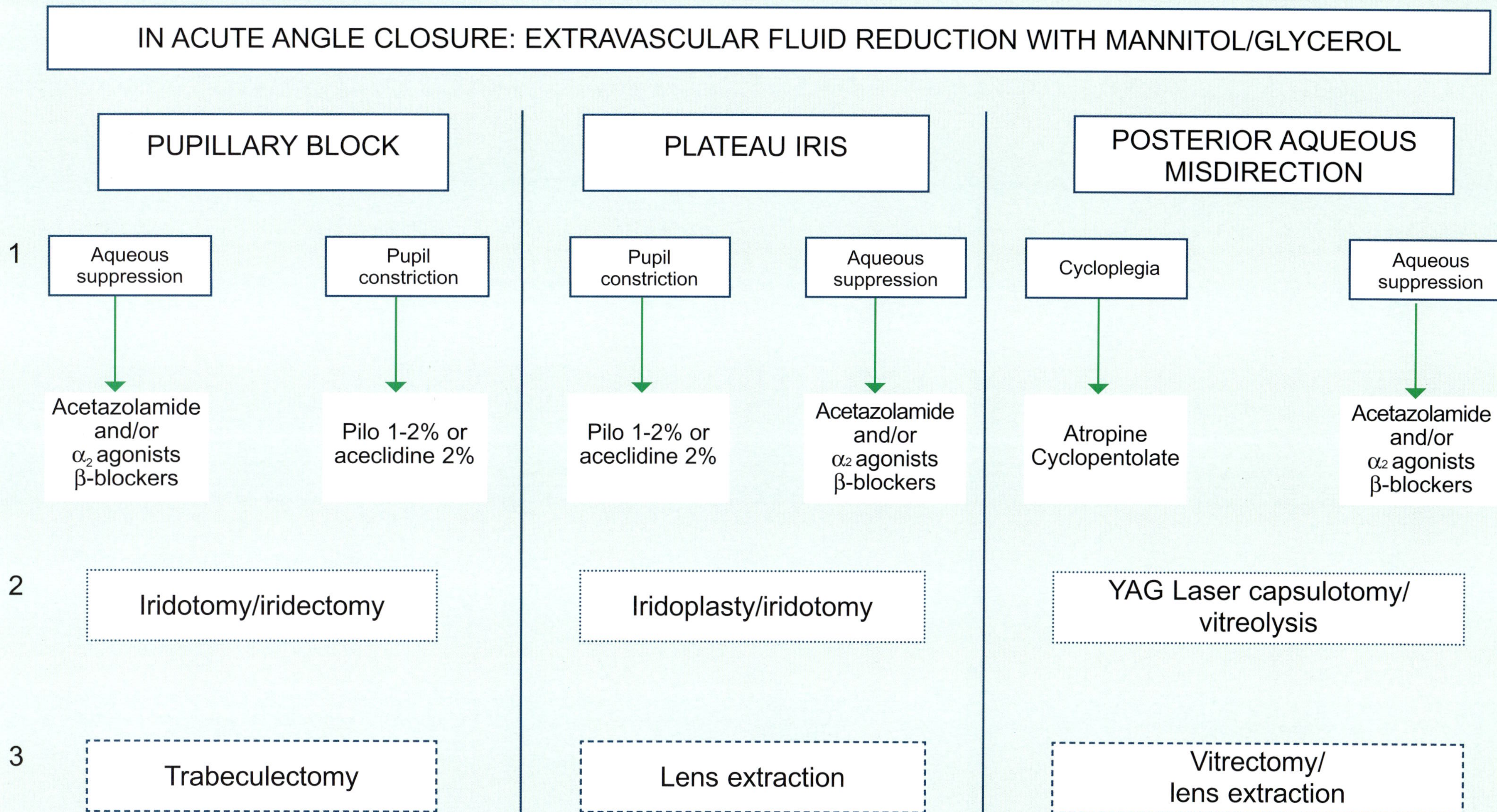

XI - MANAGEMENT ACUTE ANGLE CLOSURE GLAUCOMA WITH PUPILLARY BLOCK

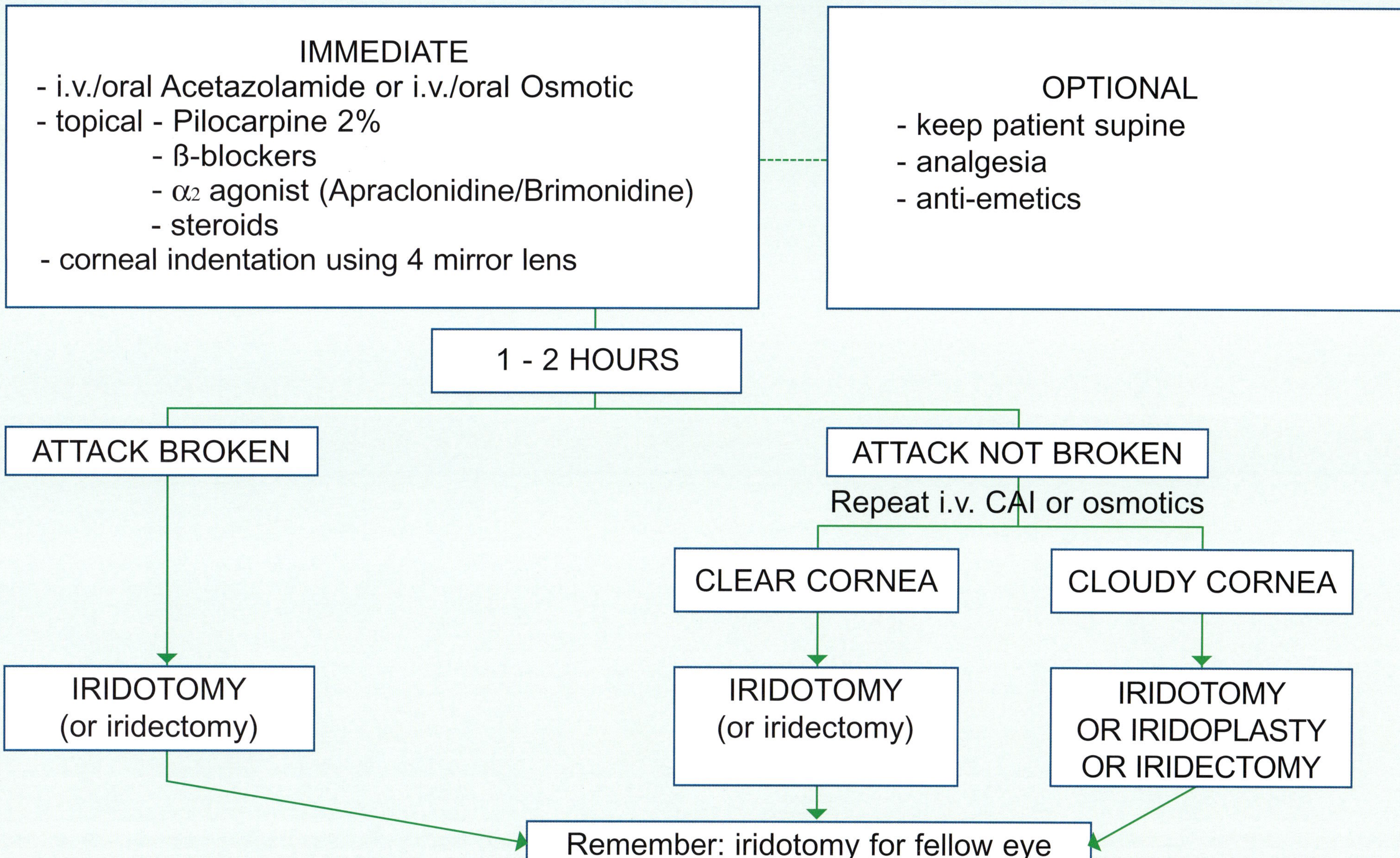

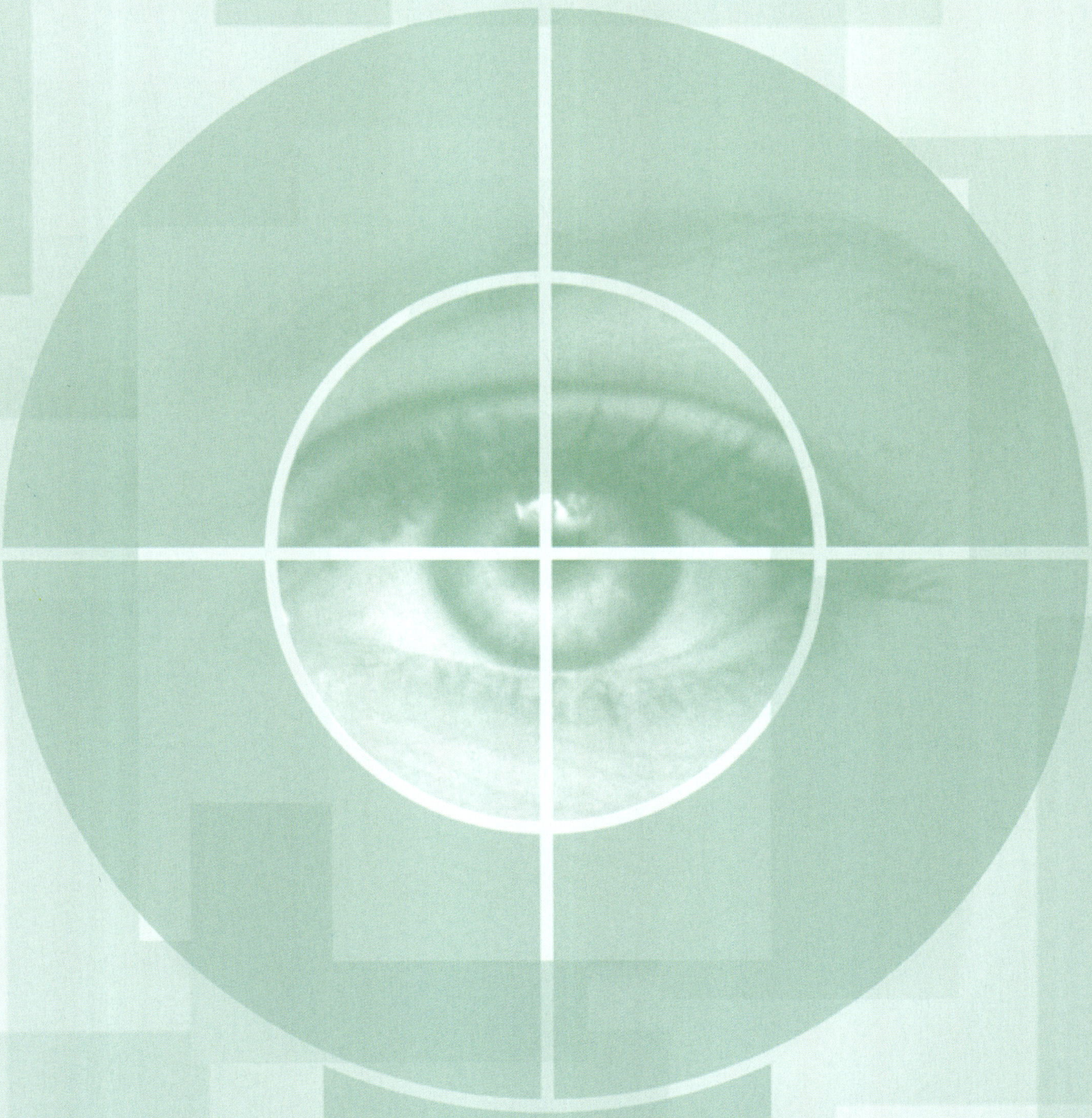

CHAPTER 1

PATIENT EXAMINATION

Normal value of intraocular pressure (IOP)
The 'normal' IOP is a statistical description of the range of IOP in the population, and is not applicable to the individual subject. There is some evidence that IOP increases by about 1 mm Hg with each decade after 40 years of age in most Western populations, although this does not appear to occur in all populations. The IOP follows a circadian cycle often with a maximum between 8 a.m. and 11 a.m. and a minimum between midnight and 2 a.m. This cycle is more dependent on the sleep cycle than the daylight cycle. The diurnal variation can be between 3 and 5 mm Hgand is wider in untreated glaucoma[1-5].

Anesthetic effects on the IOP measurement.
The IOP measurement by applanation necessitates topical anaesthesia of the cornea, which does not affect the pressure. However, in young children, topical anaesthesia is not sufficient and a general anaesthetic has to be given. The most used substances are halothane (inhaled), ketamine (intra-muscular) and chloral hydrate (oral). In general, halothane lowers the IOP, whereas ketamine can cause a transient rise in IOP. Under ketamine the IOP is usually about 4 mm Hg higher than under halothane. Oxygen given during the anaesthesia has a hypotensive effect and carbon-dioxide a hypertensive effect. Succinylcholine can produce a transitory IOP increase of about 15 mm Hg. Nitrous oxide causes a slight increase in IOP[6-9].

Normal IOP in children.
The IOP increases by about 1 mm Hg per 2 years between birth and the age of 12 years, rising from 6 to 8 mm Hg at birth to 12 ± 3 mm Hg at age 12.

Normal IOP in adults and elderly.
Normal IOP values are often based on population samples that may not be fully representative in their age distribution, as in the Framingham study where the mean age was 65 years and the mean IOP 16.5 mm Hg.

Cornea
Corneal characteristics that can affect the IOP measurements are corneal thickness, curvature and hydration[2,10-20]. The condition of the cornea should be considered both cross sectionally when comparing individuals or groups, and longitudinally when evaluating any patient. See next page.

Other artifacts
A tight collar or tie, Valsalva's manovrer, holding breath, a lid speculum or squeezing the lids can all falsely increase the IOP reading[21].

Tonometry
The principle of the method of tonometry is based on the relationship between the intraocular pressure and the force necessary to deform the natural shape of the cornea by a given amount. The deformation can be achieved by indentation, as with the Schiøtz tonometer, or by applanation, as with the Maklakoff and the Goldmann tonometers[2]. Although the pressure measured is external to the eye, the term used is "intraocular pressure"[7].

Method of measurement
The most frequently used instrument is the Goldmann applanation tonometer, mounted at the slit lamp. The method involves illumination of the biprism tonometer head with a blue light obtained using a cobalt filter and applanation of the cornea after applying topical anaesthesia and fluorescein in the tear film. The scaled knob on the side of the instrument is then turned until the hemicircle of fluorescent tear meniscus visualized thorough each prism just overlap.
Goldmann's original equation is based on the Imbert- Fick law and assumed that: the cornea had a constant radius of curvture, the rigidity was the same in all eyes, the globe was spherical, aqueous would not mave away from the AC during measurement. This adds to the expected inter and intra observer variability[20].

Other methods[22-25]:

Air-puff tonometry

The noncontact tonometer deforms the corneal apex by means of a pulsed jet of air. The exposure time is between 1 and 3 msec. Since this is 0.002 of a cardiac cycle, the ocular pulse can be a significant source of variability. Topical anathesia is not necessary. Air-puff tonometry is not recommended for evaluating patients with glaucoma.

Pneumatonometry

The sensor measures air pressure. The measurements are well correlated with those made with the Goldmann applanation tonometer, with a tendency to higher IOP estimates. It is useful in eyes with scarred, edematous and irregular cornea.

Tono-Pen

This instrument has software that automatically selects the acceptable measurements and rejects the inappropriate ones. An average of at least three good IOP measurements are determined and displayed. It is useful in patients with corneal edema or irregularities[10-13].

The relationship between CCT and different types of glaucoma is under scrutiny; in some studies a correlation between thicker corneas and OH as well as between thinner corneas and NPG were found[11,32,33,34].

INFLUENCE OF CORNEAL STATUS ON THE INTRAOCULAR PRESSURE VALUE MEASURED WITH THE GOLDMANN APPLANATION TONOMETER[26-31]

CORNEA STATUS	IOP READING		
	Erroneously high		Erroneously low
Thinner		Error Range 0.2-0.7 mmHg/10 µm	+
Thicker	+		
Edema			+
Increased power	1mmHg/3 dioptres		
Decreased power			1mmHg/3 dioptres
Astigmatism with the rule			1mmHg/4 dioptres
Astigmatism against the rule	1mmHg/4 dioptres		
Astigmatism irregular	+/-		+/-
Tear film too abundant			+
Tear film insufficient	+		
Corneal Refractive surgery*			
Lamellar cut			-/?
Radial keratotomy			-/?
Surface excimer laser (PRK)** MYOPIC			++
Intrastromal excimer laser (LASIK)**MYOPIC			++

Note: to minimize the reading errors of IOP, the biprism should be aligned to the center of the cornea. In case of high or irregular astigmatism, two measurements should be made, the first with the biprism in horizontal position and the second in vertical position and readings averaged. Measurement of IOP with a Tonopen XL (tm) may be useful in eyes with corneal surface irregularities.

* Corneal refractive surgery alters tonometry reading since it modifies thickness, curvature and structure of the cornea

** Depends on attempted correction; a precise relationship is not defined yet.

Central corneal thickness measurements are valuable:

- only to correct for Goldmann applanation IOP measurement
- if interpreted within the general variability of tonometry readings
- especially when treatment of ocular hypertension is considered
- when clinical findings do not match with IOP
- very little for management of established glaucoma
- after corneal refractive surgery

Tonography and Water Drinking

Tonography is a clinical, non invasive method for estimating the outflow facility of aqueous humor. Today it is rarely used and it has virtually disappeared from clinical pratice[3,4,14,15].

Water-drinking has been used to assess indirectly the ouflow facility. Patients are asked to drink a fixed amount of water (usually 1 liter) in a short time (usually 5 minutes) and the IOP is measured during the first hour(s). If the IOP raises substantially the test is considered positive[3,35].

IOP diurnal variations can be substantial.

IOP diurnial variations are larger in glaucoma patients.

Measurement artefacts are important variabiles.

Single IOP measurements are made during only a few seconds of a patient's day.

References

1) Martin XD. Normal intraocular pressure in man. Ophthalmologica 1992;205:57-63.
2) Fran Smith MA. Clinical exmanination of Glaucoma. In: Yanoff M, Dueker J (eds). Ophthalmology. London, Mosby 1999;12:4.1-4.3.
3) Medeiros FA, Pinheiro A, Moura FC, Leal BC, Susanna R Jr. Intraocular pressure fluctuations in medical versus surgically treated glaucomatous patients. J Ocul Pharmacol Ther 2002;18:489-498.
4) Shields RB. Textbook of Glaucoma. Baltimore, Williams & Wilkins, 1987;45-64.
5) Weber J, Koll W, Krieglstein GK. Intraocular pressure and visual field decay in chronic glaucoma. Germ J Ophthalmol 1993;2:165-169.
6) Jaafar MS, Kazi GA. Effect of oral chloral hydrate sedation on the intraocular pressure measurement. J Pediatr Ophthalmol Strabismus 1993;30:372-376.
7) Jaafar MS, Kazi GA. Normal intraocular pressure a children: a comparative study of the Perkins applanation tonometer and the pneumatonometer. J Pediatr Ophthalmol Strabismus 1993;30:284-287.
8) Epley KD, Tychsen L, Lueder GT. The effect of an eyelid speculum on intraocular pressure measurement in children. Am J Ophthalmol 2002;14:926-927.
9) Tangwiwat S, Kumphong P, Surasaraneewong S, Audchaneeyasakul L, Surachatkumthornkul T, Naksarn M, Tongkumpan P, Napachoti T. Intraocular pressure changes during general anesthesia in children, comparing no mask, undermask and laryngeal mask airway. J Med Assoc Thai 2002 85 Suppl:S975-979.
10) Doughty MJ, MLaiquzzaman M, Muller A, Oblak E, Button NF. Central corneal thickness in European (white) individuals, especially children and the ederly, and assessment of its possible importance in clinical measures of intraocular pressure. Ophthalmic Physiol Opt 2002;2:491-504.
11) Brandt JD, Beiser JA, Kass MA, Gordon MO. The ocular hypertension treatment study (OHTS) group: central corneal thickness in the ocular hypertension treatment study (OHTS). Ophthalmology 2001;108:1779-1788.
12) Hahn S, Azen S, Ying-Lai M, Varma R. Central corneal thickness in latinos. Invest Ophthalmol Vis Sci 2003;44:1508-1512.
13) Nemesure B, Wu SY, Hennis A, Leske MC. Corneal thickness and intraocular pressure in the Barbados eye studies. Arch Ophthalmol 2003;121:240-244.
14) Medeiros FA, Sample PA, Weinreb RN. Corneal thickness measurements and visual function abnormalities in ocular hypertensive patients. Am J Ophthalmol 2003;135:131-137.
15) Morgan AJ, Harper J, Hosking SL, Gilmartin B. The effect of corneal thickness and corneal curvature on pneumatonometer measurements. Curr Eye Res 2002;25:107-112.
16) Bhan A, Browning AC, Shah S, Hamilton R, Dave D, Dua HS. Effect of corneal thickness on intraocular pressure measurements with the pneumotonometer, Goldmann applanation tonometer, and Tono-Pen. Invest Ophthalmol Vis Sci 2002;43:1389-1392.
17) Bron AM, Creuzot-Garcher CP, Boutillon S, Morales C, Lewden O. Corneal thickness and intraocular pressure meaning. Invest Ophthalmol Vis Sci 1997,68:1056.
18) Ehlers N, Hansen FK, Aasved H. Biometric correlations of corneal thickness. Acta Ophthalmologica 1975;53:652-659.
19) Mark HH: Corneal curvature in applanation tonometry. Am J Ophthalmol 1993;76:223-224.
20) Whitacre MM, Stein R. Sources of error with use of Goldmann-type tonometers. Surv Ophthalmol 1993;38:1-30.
21) Brandt J. Congenital Glaucoma. In: Yanoff M. Dueker J (eds). Ophthalmology. London, Mosby 1999;12:10.2-10.3.
22) Smith DA, Trope GE. New generation portable tonometers: comparison of keta and Goldmann tonometers. Can J Ophthalmol 1989;24:308.
23) Langham ME, McCarthy E. A rapid pneumatic applanation tonometer: comparative findings and evaluation. Arch Ophthalmol 1968;79:389-499.
24) Marchini G, Babighian S, Specchia L, Perfetti S. Evaluation of the new Ocuton S tonometer. Acta Ophthalmol Scan 2002;80:167-171.
25) Iester M, Mermoud A, Achache F, Roy S. New Tonopen XL. Comparison with the Goldmann tonometer. Eye 2001;15:52-58.
26) Chatterjee A, Shah S, Bessant DA, Naroo SA, Doyle SJ. Reduction in Intraocular Pressure after Excimer Laser Photorefractive Keratectomy. Correlation with pretreatment Myopia. Ophthalmology 1997;104:355-359.
27) Cennamo G, Rosa N, La Rana A, Bianco S, Sebastiani A. Non-contact tonometry in patients that underwent photorefractive keratectomy. Ophthalmologica 1997;211:41-343.

28) Faucher A, Grégoire J, Blondeau P. Accuracy of Goldmann tonometry after refractive surgery. J Cataract Refract Surg 1997;23:832-837.
29) Levy Y, Hefetz L, Zadok D, Krakowski D, nemet P. Refractory intraocular pressure increase after photorefractive keratectomy. J Cataract Refract Surg 1997;23:539-594.
30) Schipper I, Senn P, Niesen U. Do we measure the right intraocular pressure after Excimer-Laser PRK for myopia. Klin Monatsbl Augenheilkd 1995;206:322-324.
31) Tuunanen TH, Hämäläinen P, Mali M, Oksala O, Tervo T. Effect of photorefractive keratectomy on the accuracy of pneumatonometer readings in rabbits. Invest Ophthalmol Vis Sci 1996;37:1810-1914.
32) Herdon LW, Choudhri SA, Cox T, Damji KF, Shields MB, Alligham RR. Central corneal thickness in normal, glauco matous, and ocular hypertensive eyes. Arch Ophthalmol 1997;115:1137-1141.
33) Ehlers N, Hansen FK. Central corneal thickness in low-tension glaucoma. Acta Ophthalmologica 1974;52:740-746.
34) Wolfs RC, Klaver CC, Vingerling JR, Grobbee DE, Hofman A, de Jong PT. Distribution of central corneal thickness and its association with intraocular pressure: The Rotterdam Study. Am J Ophthalmol 1997;123:767-772.
35) Diestelhorst M, Krieglstein GK. The effect of the water-drinking test on aqueous humor dynamics in healthy volunteers. Graefes Arch Clin Exp Ophthalmol 1994;232:145-147.

Gonioscopy is a fundamental part of the comprehensive eye examination[1-3] (see FC V).
Purpose of gonioscopy is to determine the topography of the anterior chamber angle. It is based on the recognition of angle landmarks, and must always consider at least the following:

a) level of iris insertion, both true and apparent
b) shape of the peripheral iris profile
c) estimated width of the angle approach
d) degree of trabecular pigmentation
e) areas of iridotrabecular apposition or synechia[4].

1.2.1 - ANATOMY

Reference landmarks

Schwalbe's line: this is a collagen condensation of the Descemet's membrane between the trabecular meshwork and the corneal endothelium and appears as a thin translucent line. Schwalbe's line may be prominent and anteriorly displaced (posterior embryotoxon) or there may be heavy pigmentation over it. Confusion between a pigmented Schwalbe's line and the trabecular meshwork may occur, particularly when the iris is convex. Indentation gonioscopy is helpful in these cases.

Trabecular Meshwork (TM): this extends posteriorly from Schwalbe's line to the scleral spur. Most difficulties concerning the examination of this region relate to the determination of features as normal or pathological, particularly pigmentation, blood vessels and iris processes.

Pigmentation: pigment is found predominantly in the posterior meshwork. It is seen in adults (rare before puberty) and is highly variable. The most common condition associated with dense pigmentation are: pseudoexfoliation syndrome, pigment dispersion syndrome, previous trauma, previous laser treatment of the iris, uveitis and acute angle-closure attack.

Blood vessels: these are often found in normal iridocorneal angles. They characteristically have a radial or circumferential orientation, have few anastomoses and do not run across the scleral spur. They can be seen most easily in subjects with blue irides. Pathological vessels are thinner, have a disordered orientation and may run across the scleral spur (neovascular membrane). Abnormal vessels are also seen in Fuch's heterochromic iridocyclitis, rubeosis and chronic anterior uveitis.

Schlemm's canal: this is not normally visible, though it may be seen if it contains blood. Blood reflux from episcleral veins may occur in cases of carotid-cavernous fistulae, Sturge Weber syndrome, venous compression, ocular hypotony, sickle cell disease or due to suction from the goniolens.

Iris processes: these are present in 1/3 of normal eyes and are frequently found in brown eyes and in youths. They follow the iris concavity and do not block the iris movements during indentation gonioscopy. When numerous and prominent they may represent a form of Axenfeld-Rieger syndrome.

Ciliary band and iris root: the iris insertion is usually at the anterior face of the ciliary body, though the site is variable. The ciliary band may be wide, as in myopia, aphakia or following trauma, or narrow or absent as in hyperopia and anterior insertion of the iris.

1.2.2 - TECHNIQUES

Gonioscopy is an essential part of the evaluation of all glaucoma patients.
There are two principal techniques for viewing the anterior chamber angle:

Direct Gonioscopy

The use of a contact goniolens like the Koeppe lens permits the light from the anterior chamber to pass through the cornea so that the angle may be viewed.

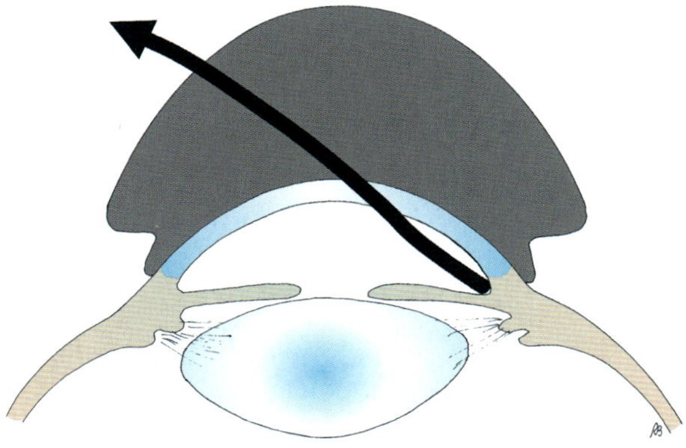

Some peculiarities of this technique are:
Patients must lie on their back
Gives a direct view of the anterior chamber angle
Good magnification
Easy orientation for the observer
Possible simultaneous comparison of both eyes
Requires high magnification whit illuminated loupes or portable slit-lamp
Angle view possible with direct ophthalmoscope by dialing high plus lens

Indirect Gonioscopy

The light from the anterior chamber is made to exit via a mirror built into a contact glass.

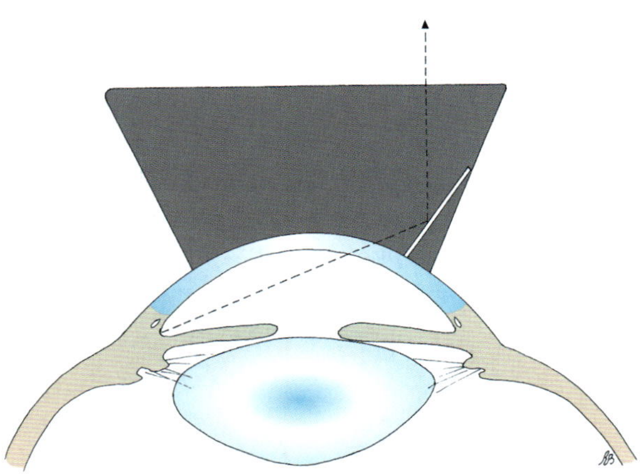

Some peculiarities of this technique are:
Patient must be at the slit lamp
Indirect view of the anterior chamber angle
Faster than direct gonioscopy during routine ophthalmological exam
It can be used to see the fundus (using the central part of the lens) at the slit lamp.
Inability to compare the two eyes simultaneously

The most common Gonioscopy lenses:

Direct
Koeppe (contact fluid required)
Layden (sized for infants; contact fluid required)
Worst

Indirect
Posner or Zeiss or Sussman 4 mirror (contact fluid not required)
Goldmann lens, 1 to 4 mirrors (contact fluid required)
CGA 1.4© Lasag (contact fluid required)

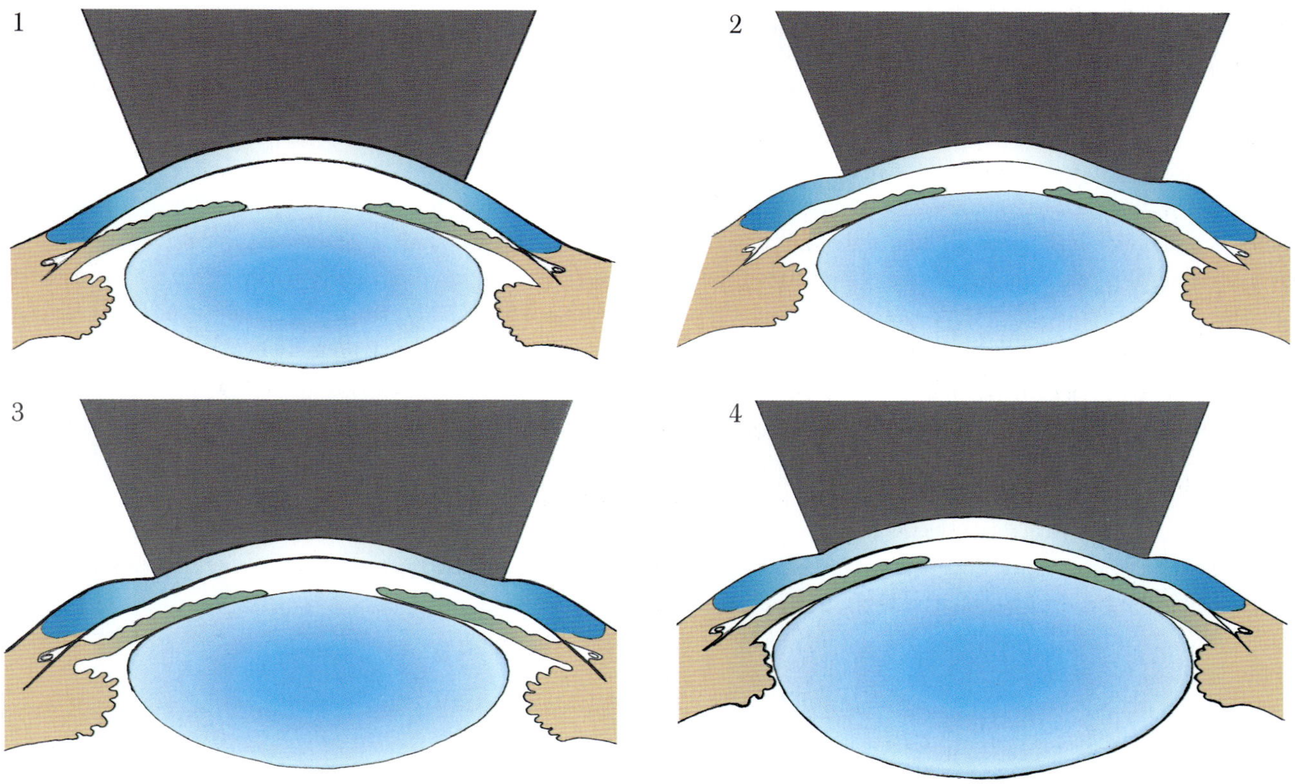

Fig. 1
Dynamic indentation gonioscopy. When no angle structure is directly visible before indentation, angle-closure can be synechial or appositional or optical, the latter being apparent closure due to the curvature of the peripheral iris (1). If during indentation the iris moves peripherally backwards and the angle recess widens (2), the picture in (1) is to be interpreted as appositional closure and a suspicion of relative pupillary block is raised (2). When during indentation the angle widens but iris strands remain attached to the angle outer wall (3), the picture in (1) is to be interpreted as synechial closure. A large and\or anteriorly displaced lens causes the iris to move only slightly and evenly backwards during indentation (4) making the lens a likely component of angle-closure.

Dynamic Indentation by 4-mirror Gonioscopy
For this technique the ideal 4 mirror lens has a flat anterior surface and a posterior surface with a radius of curvature of 7.7 mm. Since this is longer than the average corneal radius of curvature it allows corneal contact via the tear film without the need for a contact medium. When gentle pressure is applied by the lens on the centre of the cornea, the aqueous humour is pushed back. When the iris lies in contact with the trabecular meshwork in appositional angle-closure, the angle can be re-opened. If there is adhesion between the iris and the meshwork, as in goniosynechia, that portion of angle remains closed (Fig. 1). This technique is specifically useful where the curvature of the iris surface is convex, making it difficult to recognise the different angle structures listed in 1.2.1.

Dynamic indentation gonioscopy should be performed in **all cases being evaluated for glaucoma**.
When pupillary block is the prevalent mechanism the iris becomes peripherally concave during indentation. In iris plateau configuration this iris concavity will not be extended by indentation to the extreme periphery, which is a sign of anteriorly placed ciliary body or iris root. When the lens has a role, indentation causes the iris to move only slightly backwards, retaining a convex profile (Fig. 1).

Dynamic indentation gonioscopy is extremely useful to **differentiate optical from either appositional or synechial closure**, as well as for measuring the extent of angle-closure.

Gonioscopy technique without indentation

With indirect Goldmann-type lenses it is preferable to start by viewing the superior angle, which often appears narrower, and then to continue rotating the mirror, maintaining the same direction in each examination. The anterior surface of the lens should be kept perpendicular to the observation axis so that the appearance of the angle structure is not changed as the examination proceeds. The four quadrants are examined by a combination of slit-lamp movements and prism rotation.

In case of a narrow approach, it is possible to improve the visualization of the angle recess by having the patient rotate the globes towards the mirror being used.

Problems

Related to the technique

The most widely used technique is indirect gonioscopy where the angle is viewed in a mirror of the lens. The position of the globe is influential. If the patient looks in the direction opposite of the mirror the angle appears narrower and viceversa.
A second pitfall is related to the degree of pressure of the lens against the cornea and especially occurs when the diameter of the lens is smaller than the corneal diameter (as with the small Goldmann lens, the Posner or the Zeiss lenses). This effect is useful for indentation or dynamic gonioscopy with the Posner or Zeiss lenses; inadvertent pressure over the cornea however, will push back the iris, and gives an erroneously wide appearance to the angle. With the Goldman lens indentation is transmitted to the periphery of the cornea and narrows the angle.

Related to the anatomy

Recognition of angle structures may be impaired by variations in the anterior segment structures like poor pigmentation, iris convexity or existence of pathological structures. The examiner should be familiar with all the anatomical structures of the angle: Schwalbe's line, trabecular meshwork, scleral spur, ciliary band and iris.

Pharmacological mydriasis

Dilation of the pupil with topical or systemic drugs can trigger iridotrabecular contact or pupillary block, eventually leading to angle-closure. Angle-closure attacks can occur, even bilaterally, in patients treated with systemic parasympatholytics before, during or after abdominal surgery and has been reported with a serotonergic appetite suppressant.
Although pharmacological mydriasis with topical tropicamide and neosynephrine is safe in the general population even in eyes with very narrow approach, in occasional patients raised IOP and an angle occlusion can be observed.
Theoretically, although any psychoactive drugs have the potential to cause angle-closure, it is unlikely that pre-treatment gonioscopy findings alone are of help to rule out such risk. In eyes with narrow angles, it makes sense to repeat gonioscopy and tonometry after initiation of treatment. Prophylactic laser iridotomy needs to be evaluated against the risks of angle-closure or of withdrawal of the systemic treatment. (See Chapter 2 - 4). None of these drugs is contraindicated per se in open-angle glaucoma.
Ciliochoroidal detachment with bilateral angle-closure has been reported after oral sulfa drugs.
Since patients most commonly have mixed components of angle-closure, gonioscopic appearances are seldom clear-cut as far as determining the etiology.
The visualization during gonioscopy of the ciliary processes through the undilated pupil is a sign of forward displacement of the iris and of the anterior lens surface, associated with anterior rotation of the ciliary body.

1.2.3 - GRADING

The use of a grading system for gonioscopy is highly desirable[2,5,6]. It stimulates the observer to use a systematic approach in evaluating angle anatomy, it allows comparison of findings at different times in the same patients, or to classify different patients.
A grading method is also very helpful to record the gonioscopy findings and should always be used on patients' charts.
The Spaeth gonioscopy grading system is the only descriptive method including all the parameters described above (chapter 1.2.1)[2]. Other grading systems are useful though less specific. There are several gonioscopy classification systems; we list the most widespread.

Slit lamp-grading of peripheral AC depth - the Van Herick method[7]

Grade 0 represents iridocorneal contact.
A space between iris and corneal endothelium of $< 1/4$ corneal thickness, is a grade I.
When the space is $\geq 1/4 < 1/2$ corneal thickness the grade is II.
A grade III is considered not occludable, with an irido/endothelial distance $\geq 1/2$ corneal thickness.
This technique is based on the use of corneal thickness as a unit measure of the depth of the anterior chamber at furtherest periphery. This method is very useful if a goniolens is not available[7,8].

The Spaeth classification

Insertion of iris root

1

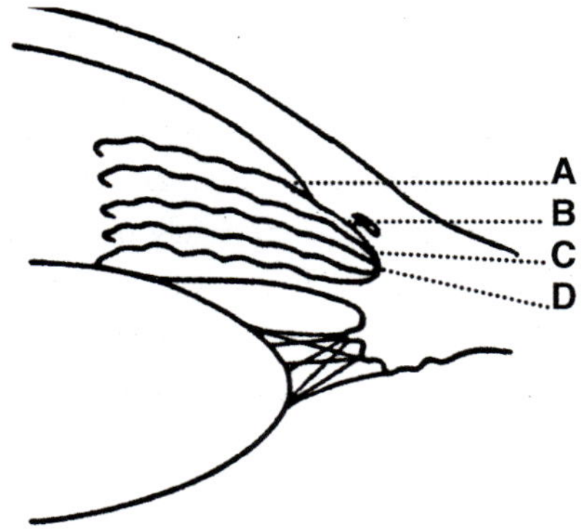

A	Anterior to Schwalbe's line
B	Behind Schwalbe's line
C	On the Scleral Spur
D	Behind the Scleral Spur
E	On the Ciliary Band

Angular width of angle recess

2

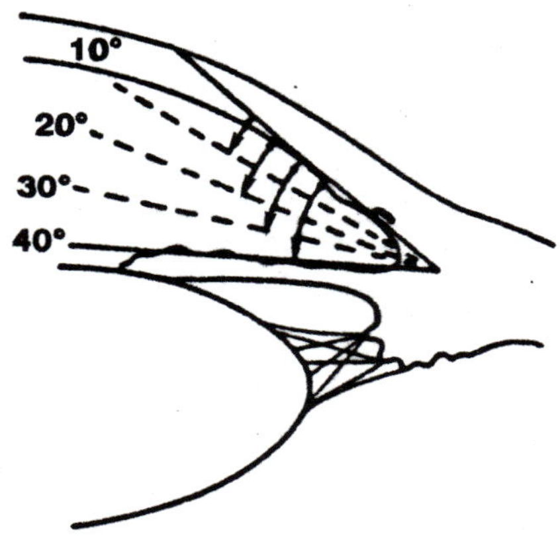

Slit	
10°	narrow
20°	narrow
30°	wide
40°	wide

Configuration of the peripheral iris

3

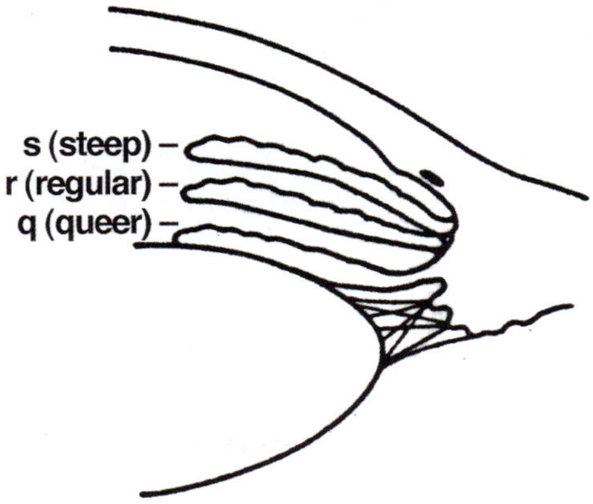

s	steep, anteriorly convex
r	regular
q	queer, anteriorly concave

The Shaffer - Etienne classification

0 -	No structures visible	closed-angle
1 -	Schwalbe line visible	closure possible
2 -	Schwalbe line and trabeculum meshwork visible, but scleral spur not visible	narrow
3 -	Scleral spur visible	closure impossible
4 -	All the structures visible from the Schwalbe line to the ciliary band	closure impossible

1.2.4 - ULTRASOUND BIOMICROSCOPY

Ultrasound biomicroscopy (U.B.M.) of the anterior segment allows accurate visualization of the iris, iris root, corneoscleral junction, ciliary body, lens[9-13].

With this technique it is possible to elucidate the mechanism of angle-closure in almost every patient. Due to its limited availability and costs however, ultrasound biomicroscopy is usually applied to cases which are most difficult to interpret.

References

1) Palmberg P. Gonioscopy. In: Ritch R, Shields MB, Krupin T (eds). The Glaucomas. St. Louis, Mosby, 1996;455-469.
2) Spaeth GL. The normal development of the human chamber angle: a new system of descriptive grading. Trans Ophthalmol Soc UK 1971;91:709-739.
3) Alward WLM. Color atlas of gonioscopy. London, Mosby, 1994.
4) Forbes M. Gonioscopy with corneal indentation: a method for distinguish between appositional closure and synechial closure. Arch Ophthalmol 1966;76:488-492.
5) Kolker AE, Hetherington J. Beker-Shaffer's diagnosis and therapy of the glaucomas. St Louis, Mosby, 1995.
6) Scheie HG. Width and pigmentation of the angle of the anterior chamber: a system of grading by gonioscopy. Arch Ophthalmol 1957;58:510-514.
7) Van Herick W, Shaffer RN, Schwartz A. Estimation of width of the angle of the anterior chamber: incidence and significance of the narrow angle. Am J Ophthalmol 1969;68:626-632.
8) Congdon NG, Spaeth GL, Augsburger J, Klanenik J Jr, Patel K, Hunter DG. A proposed simple method for measurement in the anterior chamber angle. Ophthalmology 1999;106:2161-2167.
9) Fran Smith M, Doyle WJ. Clinical examination of Glaucoma. In: Yanoff M, Duker JS (eds). London, Mosby, 1999;12:4.9.
10) Pavlin CJ, Ritch R, Foster FS. Ultrasound biomicroscopy in plateau iris syndrome. Am J Ophthalmol 1992;113:390-395.
11) Riley SF, Nairn JP, Maestre FA, Smith TJ. Analysis of the anterior chamber angle by gonioscopy and by ultrasound biomicroscopy. Int Ophthalmol Clin 1994;34:271-282.
12) Marchini G, Pagliarusco A, Toscano A, Tosi R, Brunelli C, Bonomi L. Ultrasound biomicroscopic and conventional ultrasonographic study of ocular dimensions in primary angle-closure glaucoma. Ophthalmology 1998;105:2091-2098.
13) Ishikawa H, Liebmann JM, Ritch R. Quantitative assessment of the anterior segment using ultrasound biomicroscopy. Curr Opin Ophthalmol 2000;11:133-139.

1.3 - OPTIC NERVE HEAD AND RETINAL NERVE FIBER LAYER

The identification of structural, contour and color changes is best done stereoscopically. The pupil should be dilated whenever possible to facilitate the exam. Two methods allow for time-efficient and inexpensive stereoscopic examination of the posterior pole:

- indirect fundus lens (78D or 90D) at the slit-lamp
- direct fundus lens (central part of Goldmann and Zeiss 4-mirror, Hruby) at the slit-lamp

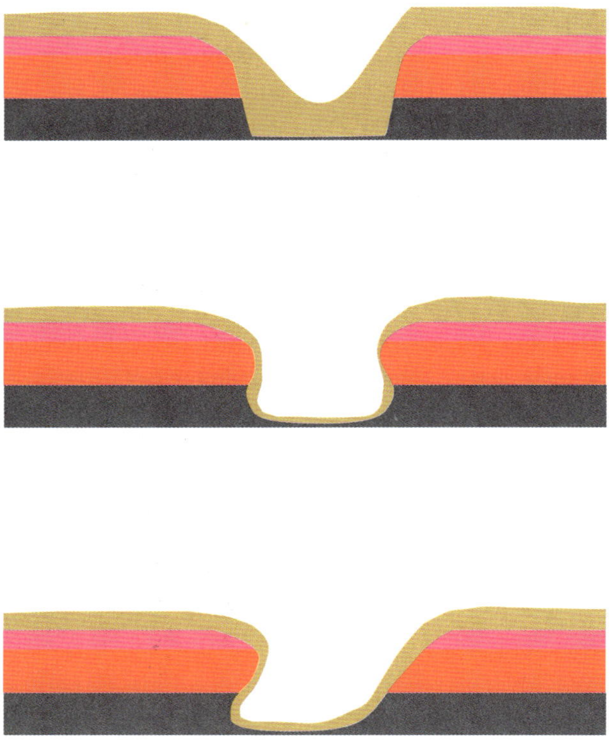

Fig. 1
Different optic nerve head contours: A) normal ONH, B) glaucomatous ONH, C) tilted ONH.

The direct ophthalmoscope can give three-dimensional information using parallax movements. It is essential to select a spot size with a diameter smaller than the diameter of the disc. This is to avoid light spreading from the peripapillary retina altering the colour appearance of the rim.
The evaluation of the optic nerve head (ONH) and retinal nerve fiber layer (RNFL) may be divided into 2 parts:

1.3.1 - Qualitative

a) contour of the neuroretinal rim
b) optic disc hemorrhages
c) parapapillary atrophy
d) bared circumlinear vessels
e) appearance of the retinal nerve fibre layer

1.3.2 - Quantitative

a) optic disc size (vertical disc diameter)
b) cup/disc ratio (vertical)
c) rim/disc ratio
d) retinal nerve fiber layer height (RNFLH)

1.3.1.a - Contour of the neuroretinal rim

With intact nerve fibers the contour of the rim depends on the shape of the optic disc canal (Fig. 1).
The disc is usually slightly vertically oval. Black subjects often have larger discs as a result of a greater vertical disc diameter[1].
In normal discs with small cups the neuroretinal rim is at least as thick at the 12 and 6 o'clock positions as elsewhere and usually thickest (83% of eyes) in the infero-temporal sector, followed by the supero-temporal, nasal and then temporal sectors (I.S.N.T.)[2]. This pattern is less marked in larger discs, in which the rim is distributed more evenly around the edge of the disc (Fig. 2a, 2b).
Optic cups are on average horizontally oval. However, large physiological cups in large discs tend to be more round than horizontally oval and the more vertically oval discs tend toward having a more vertically oval cup.
Cupping tends to be symmetrical between the two eyes, the comparative vertical cup/disc ratio being within 0.2 in over 96% of normal subjects.
Glaucoma is characterized by progressive thinning of the neuroretinal rim. The pattern of loss of rim varies and may take the form of diffuse thinning, localized notching, or both in combination (fig. 2b). Thinning of the rim, while occuring in all disc sectors, is generally greatest at the inferior and superior poles, leading to a loss of the physiological rim shape so that the infero-temporal rim is no longer the thickest[3-7].
The optic cup often enlarges in all directions, but usually the enlargement occurs predominantly in the vertical direction, as a result of rim loss at the poles (Fig. 2b).

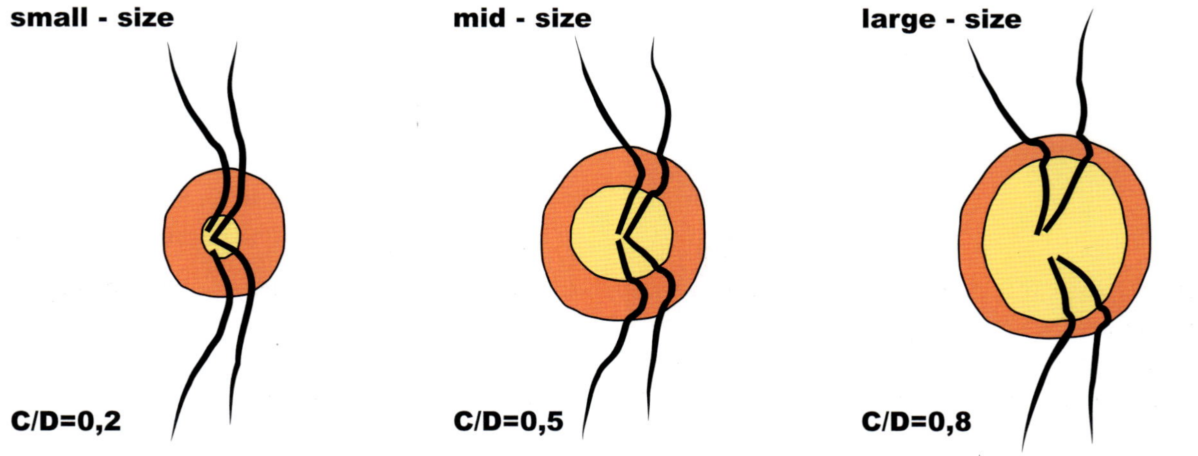

Fig. 2a (above)
Optic nerve heads with different disc area but with the same rim area and same retinal nerve fiber number: small size disc (disc area less than 2 mm^2 and C/D=0.2), mid size disc (disc area between 2 and 3 mm^2, C/D=0.5) and large disc (disc area greater than 3 mm^2 and C/D=0.8).

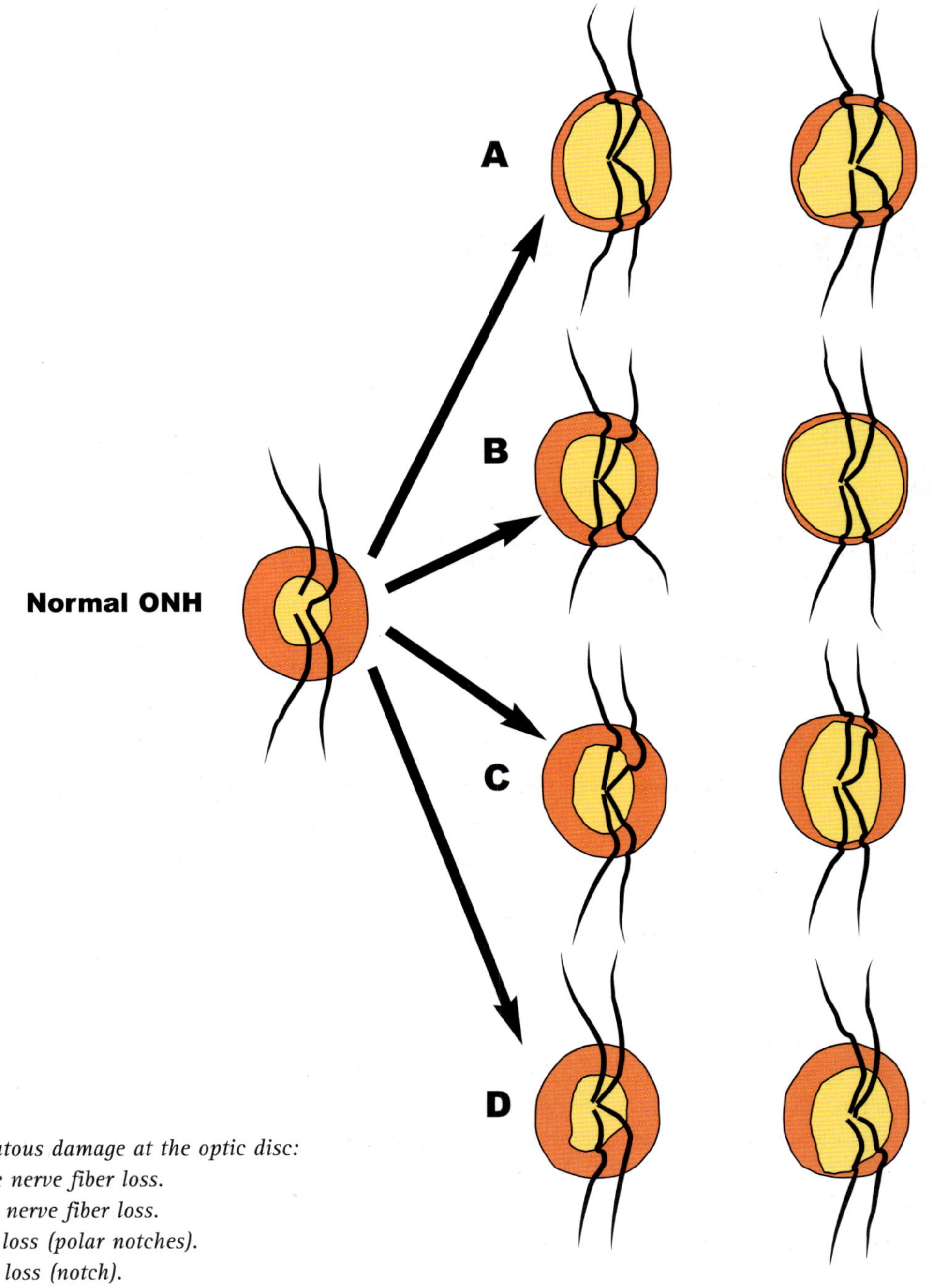

Fig. 2b
Progression of glaucomatous damage at the optic disc:
A) Localized and diffuse nerve fiber loss.
B) Diffuse or concentric nerve fiber loss.
C) Localized nerve fiber loss (polar notches).
D) Localized nerve fiber loss (notch).

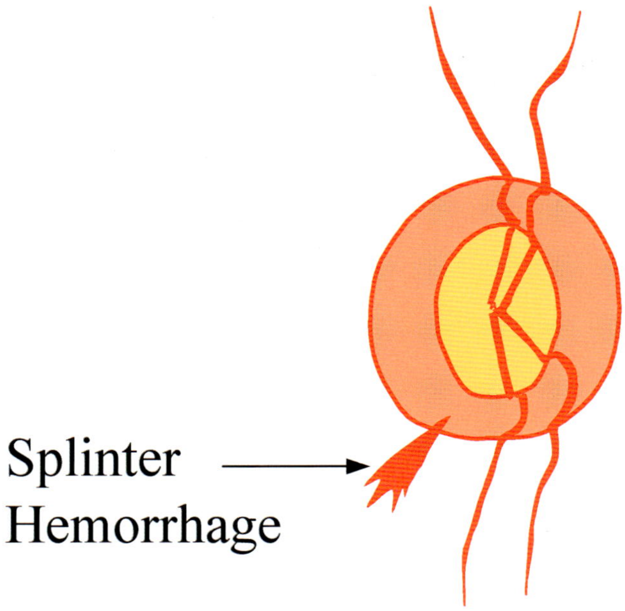

Fig. 3
Optic disc hemorrhage.

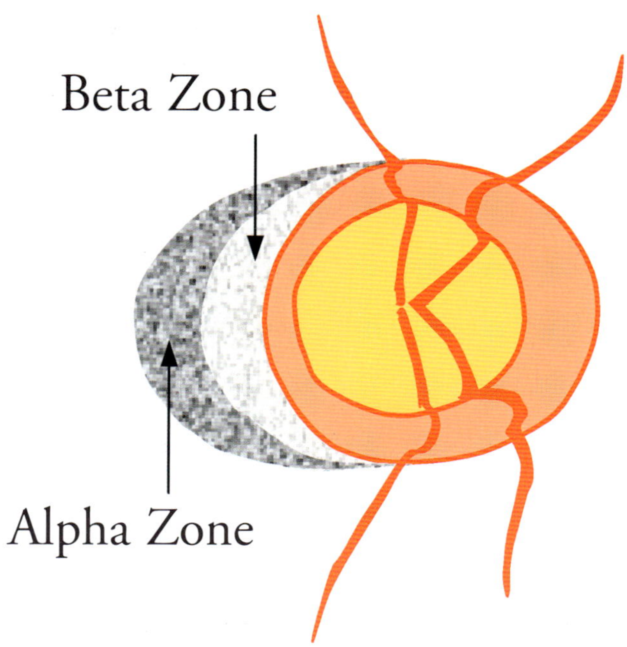

Fig. 4
ONH with parapapillary atrophy: Alpha dystrophy is located peripheral to beta dystrophy, characterized by irregular hypopigmentation and hyperpigmentation; Beta dystrophy is adjacent to the optic disc edge, outer to the Elshnig rim, with visible sclera and visible large choroidal vessels.

1.3.1.b - Optic disc hemorrhages

The prevalence of small hemorrhages related to the optic disc has been estimated at 0 to 0.21% in the normal population and 2.2 to 4.1% in glaucomatous patients; they may be more common in normal-tension glaucoma (up to 40%). Since the prevalence of disc hemorrhage is low in the normal population, their presence is very likely to be pathological, especially if recurring. It is a sign of local vascular damage[8,9] (Fig. 3).

1.3.1.c - Parapapillary atrophy[10-12]

A temporal crescent of parapapillary atrophy is common (80% in the normal population). However, the frequency and area covered increases in glaucoma. Parapapillary atrophy is least frequent in normal eyes in the nasal disc sector. The site of the largest area of atrophy tends to correspond with the part of the disc with most neuroretinal rim loss. The extent of atrophy may be greater in NPG. Because some degree of atrophy is present in many normal eyes, a large area of atrophy should be regarded as an extra clue, rather than as a definite sign of local vascular damage associated with glaucoma (Fig. 4).

1.3.1.d - Acquired baring of circumlinear vessels

An early sign of acquired rim thinning is a circumlinear vessel becoming bared. A circumlinear vessel is a small arteriole or vein that lies superficially on the neuroretinal rim, at its inner edge, and leaves the disc towards the macula; at least one is present in about 50% of eyes. As the rim narrows the loss of tissue leaves this vessel isolated, or 'bared'. It may then remain superficial or come to lie on the inner slope of the rim or on the cup floor (Fig. 5).

1.3.1.e - Appearance of the retinal nerve fibre layer

The nerve fibre layer (NFL) is best seen with a 78D or 90D lens or a contact lens at the slit lamp with a bright, rectangular, green light. The fibre bundles are seen as silver striations. From about two discs diameters from the disc the NFL thins and feathers-out. Slit-like, groove-like, or spindle-shaped apparent defects, narrower than the retinal vessels, are seen in the normal fundus. The NFL becomes less visible with age, and is more difficult to see in lightly pigmented fundi.

Defects are best seen within two disc diameters of the disc. Wedge and slit defects (wider than retinal vessels) are more apparent in early disease, when there is little generalized thinning of the NFL, and are seen as dark bands extending from the optic disc. Generalized thinning of the NFL, with a loss of brightness and density of striations, is a difficult sign to objectively confirm. When the NFL is thinned the blood vessel walls are sharp and the vessels appear to stand out in relief against a matt back-

Fig. 5
A) Cirumlinear vessel,
B) Bared circumlinear vessel

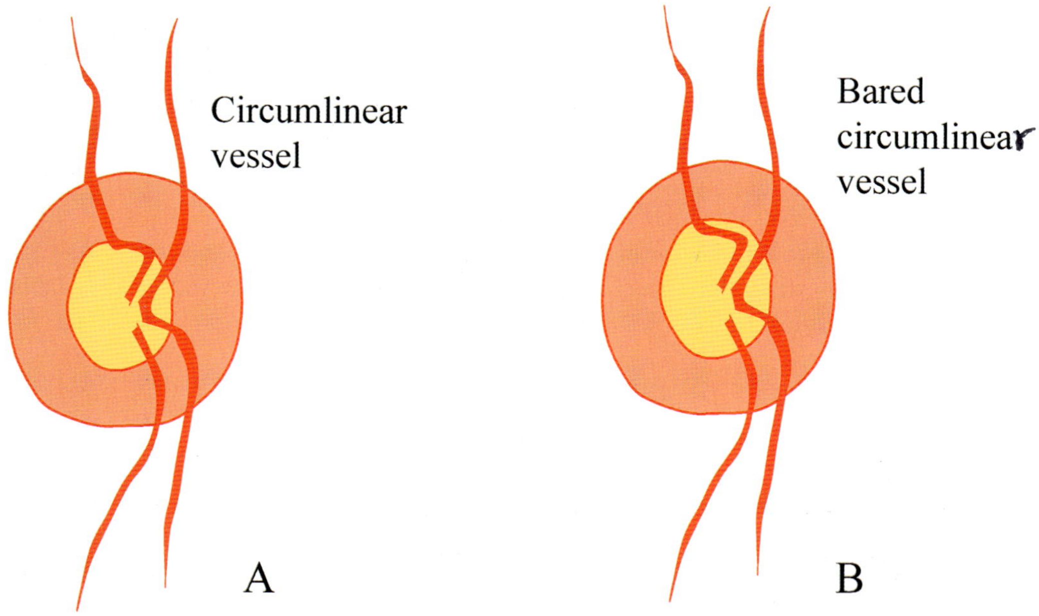

ground. The initial abnormality in glaucoma may be either diffuse thinning or localized defects. Since the prevalence of true NFL defects is < 3% in the normal population, their presence is very likely to be pathological[13-18].

1.3.2.a - Optic disc size (vertical disc diameter)

The thickness of the rim and, conversely, the size of the cup varies physiologically with the overall size of the disc[19]. The size of optic discs varies greatly in the population.

Disc size is related to refractive error, being usually smaller in hyperopes than in myopes. Discs in highly myopic eyes above 7 diopters are harder to interpret.

The vertical diameter of the optic disc can be measured at the slit lamp using a contact or a condensing lens. The slit beam should be coaxial with the observation axis; a narrow beam is used to measure the disc height using the white scleral ring as a reference landmark. The magnification corrections needed vary with the optical dimensions of the eye and with the lens used for measurement. The measured or estimated ONH size should be written in the chart.

Magnification correction factors			
Type of lens		Lim CS et al[20]	Manufacturer's data
Volk	60 D	0.88	0.92
	78 D	1.11	1.15
	90 D	1.33	1.39
Nikon	60 D	1.03	1.02
	90 D	1.63	1.54
Haag-Streit Goldmann		-	1.14

1.3.2.b - Cup/disc ratio (CDR)

The decimal value obtained by dividing the cup diameter with the disc diameter. The closer the value is to 1, the worse the damage. The vertical cup/disc ratio is a better measure of deviation from normal than the horizontal ratio, because early neuroretinal rim loss occurs preferentially at the upper and lower poles of the disc[21].

A difference in cup/disc ratio between eyes with equal overall optic disc size is suggestive of tissue loss and therefore is highly suspicious of acquired damage. Expressing the size of a cup as a cup/disc ratio (C/D or CDR) is of limited value unless the actual size of the disc is known. A CDR > 0.65 is found in less than 5% of the normal population (Fig. 2a).

1.3.2.c - Rim/disc ratio (RDR)

The fractional decimal value obtained dividing the rim thickness by the disc diameter. The closer the value is to 1, the better the optic disc appearance. It can be calculated as vertical diameters as for the cup/disc ratio but obviously with the opposite meaning, as rim area/disc area ratio (RDR or R/D). This latter can also be calculated for each degree of the optic disc as a sector index of a healthy disc.

1.3.2.d - Retinal Nerve Fiber Layer Height (RNFLH)

The thickness of the RNFL depends on disc area, age, stage of the glaucomatous damage. It has been shown that vertical polar sectors were thicker than nasal and temporal. It was also shown that RNFL height in normal was thicker than in glaucomatous subjects[16,22].

1.3.3 - RECORDING OF THE OPTIC NERVE HEAD (ONH) FEATURES

Colour disc photos are useful for patient documentation.
Colour photography with a 15° field gives optimal magnification.
Stereoscopic photographs are the preferred method. Pseudo-stereoscopic photos are also acceptable.
New systems for the ONH assessment, using alternative technologies, are being evaluated for reproducibility, specificity and sensitivity, although very few are currently available to the general ophthalmologist due to their cost (see Ch. 1.3.4).
Drawings are better than nothing if a fundus camera is not available.
Recording of the nerve fibre layer (NFL) features.
The photographic methods require specialized processing of film. Patients must have clear media and photography of lightly coloured fundi are more difficult. The technique is available in some centres, though their use in routine clinical work is limited.
New systems for NFL assessment, using alternative technologies, are being evaluated for reproducibility, specificity and sensitivity, although currently very few are available to the general ophthalmologist due to their cost (see Ch. 1.3.4).

1.3.4 - IMAGING IN GLAUCOMA

Although clinical examination still remains the most important method of assessing the ONH for glaucomatous damage, several imaging devices are now available, allowing quantitative measurements of nerve structure. This may aid clinical management[23].
These include confocal scanning laser ophthalmoscopy (e.g. Heidelberg Retina Tomograph (HRT)), scanning laser polarimetry (e.g. GDx), optical coherence tomography (e.g. OCT) and retinal thickness analyzer (e.g. RTA). Other methods of documentation of structure (e.g. stereo disc photography) are also widely used. In using these machines, accuracy and reproducibility of measurement is important, as well as the ability to discriminate between healthy and glaucomatous subjects, now very limited in early disease.

> It must be emphasized that the process of categorising patients by means of imaging device measurements is not the same as diagnosis. Diagnosis must also integrate all the other available information about the patient, including clinical assessment of the ONH and RNFL, visual field and risk factors including IOP, age and family history.
> In the future, with greater clinical information being provided by optic disc measurement and with the cost of the instruments declining, the clinical use of these devices is likely to expand.

1.3.4.1 - HRT

The Heidelberg Retina Tomograph is a confocal scanning laser which uses a 670nm light source and can assess the optic nerve head by creating a threedimensional image[24-26].

1.3.4.2 - GDX

The nerve fiber layer analyzer is a scanning laser polarimeter which uses a 780 nm polarized light source and can quantify the retinal nerve fiber layer thickness by measuring the retardation of the reflected light[27-29].

1.3.4.3 - OCT

The Optical Coherence Tomograph is a laser scanning interpherometer which can quantify the retinal structure by measuring the retardation of the reflected light[30-32].

1.3.4.4 - RTA

The Retinal Thckness Analyzer measures the distance between the vitreoretinal interface and the pigment epithelium using a 543 nm laser source[33-34].

1.3.5 - ONH APPEARANCES AND CLINICAL TYPES OF GLAUCOMA

Optic disc appearance has been used to divide POAG (HPG and NPG) into different groups. Each ophthalmologist may or may not elect to use this further sub-division.
ONH features have been used to identify a variety of POAG subtypes. However, a clear separation between these types of glaucoma is usually lacking.
Features that in some studies are more common in normal pressure glaucoma (NPG) include[35-41]:

<u>Optic disc:</u>

- localized rim damage (notch) early in the course
- flat disc excavation (no laminar excavation)
- splinter hemorrhage (often)
- peripapillary chorioretinal atrophy
- narrowing of retinal arteries

<u>Retinal Nerve Fiber Layer:</u>

- localized loss

It is unlikely for ONH findings alone to be pathognonomic of a specific type of glaucoma[37,41].

1.3.6 - PROGRESSION OF DAMAGE

Imaging is likely to play a role in the future for longitudinal follow-up[42,43]. Ophthalmoscopy techniques have also proved to be clinically useful for disease staging and for semiquantitative longitudinal evaluation of the disc[44-48].
Confirmed worsening of ONH or RNFL parameters is a strong sign of glaucoma progression.

References

1) Tsai CS, Zangwill L, Gonzalez C, Irak I, Garden V, Hoffman R, Weinreb RN. Ethnic differences in optic nerve head topography. J Glaucoma 1995;4:248-257.
2) Jonas JB, Gusek GC, Naumann GOH. Optic disc morphometry in chronic open-angle glaucoma. I. Morphometric intrapapillary characteristic. Graefe's Arch Clin Exp Ophthalmol 1988;226:522-530.
3) Tuulonen A, Airaksinen PJ. Initial glaucomatous optic disk and retinal nerve fiber layer abnormalities and their progression. Am J Ophthalmol 1991;111:485-490.
4) Quigley HA. II Changes in the appearance of the optic disk. Surv Ophthalmol 1985;30:117-126.
5) Pederson JE, Anderson DR. The mode of progressive disc cupping in ocular hypertension and glaucoma. Arch Ophthalmol 1980;98:490-495.
6) Zeyen TG, Caprioli J. Progression of disc and field damage in early glaucoma. Arch Ophthalmol 1993;111:62-65.
7) Spaeth GL. Developmant of glaucomatous changes of the optic nerve. In: Varma R, Spaeth GL, Parker KW (eds). The optic nerve in glaucoma. Philadelphia, JB Lippincott, 1993.
8) Gordon J, Piltz-Seymour JR. The significance of optic disc hemorrhages in glaucoma. J Glaucoma 1997;6:62-64.
9) Drance SM. Disc hemorrhages in the glaucomas. Surv Ophthalmol 1989;93:853-857.
10) Primrose J. Early signs of the glaucomatous disc. Br J Ophthalmol 1971;55:820-825.
11) Nervaz J, Rockwood EJ, Anderson DR. The configuration of peripapillary tissue in unilateral glaucoma. Arch Ophthalmol 1988;106:901-903.
12) Jonas JB, Nguyen NX, Gusek GC, Naumann GOH. Parapapillary chorioretinal atrophy in normal and glaucomatous eyes. I. Morphometric data. Invest Ophthalmol Vis Sci 1989;30:908.
13) Airaksinen PJ, Tuulonen A, Alanko HI. Rate and pattern of neuroretinal rim area decrease in ocular hypertension and glaucoma. Arch Ophthalmol 1992;110:206-210.
14) Hoyt WF, Schlicke B, Eckelhoff RJ. Funduscopic appearance of a nerve fiber bundle defect. Br J Ophthalmol 1972;56:577-583.
15) Hoyt WF, Frisèn L, Newman NM. Funduscopy of nerve fiber layer defects in glaucoma. Invest Ophthalmol Vis Sci 1973;12:814-829.
16) Iester M, Courtright P, Mikelberg FS. Retinal nerve fiber layer height in high-tension glaucoma and healthy eyes. J Glaucoma 1998;7:1-7.
17) Jonas JB, Nguyen NX, Naumann GOH. The retinal nerve fiber layer in normal eyes. Ophthalmology1989;96:627.
18) Airaksinen PJ, Drance SM, Douglas GR, Schultzer M, Wijsman K. Visual field and retinal nerve fiber layer comparisons in glaucoma. Arch Ophthalmol 1985;103:205-207.
19) Iester M, Mikelberg FS, Drance SM. The effect of optic disc size on diagnostic precision with the Heidelberg Retina Tomograph. Ophthalmology 1997;104:545-548.
20) Lim CS, O'Brien C, Bolton NM. A simple clinical method to measure the optic disc size in glaucoma. J Glaucoma 1996;5:241-245.
21) Gloster J. Quantitative relationship between cup ping of the optic disc and visual field loss in chronic simple glaucoma. Br J Ophthalmol 1978;62:665-669.
22) Caprioli J. The contour of the juxtapapillary nerve fiber layer in glaucoma. Ophthalmology 1990;97:358-366.
23) Mardin CY, Junemann AGM. The diagnostic value of optic nerve imaging in early glaucoma. Curr Opin Ophthalmol 2001;12:100-104.
24) Iester M, Mardin CY, Budde WM, Junemann AG, Hayler JK, Jonas JB. Discriminant analysis formulas of optic nerve head parameters measured by Confocal Scanning Laser Tomography. J Glaucoma. 2002;11:97-104.
25) Chauhan BC, McCormick TA, Nicolela MT, LeBlanc RP. Optic disc and visual field changes in a prospective logitudinal study of patients with glaucoma. Arch Ophthalmol 2001;119:1492-1499.
26) Wollstein G, Garway-Heath DF, Hitchings RA: Identification of early glaucoma cases with the scanning laser ophthalmoscope. Ophthalmology 1998;105:1557-1563.
27) Hollo G, Suveges I, Nagymihaly A, vargha P. Scanning laser polarimetry of the retinal nerve fiber layer in primary open-angle and capsular glaucoma. Br J Ophthalmol 1997;81:857-861.
28) Greenfield DS, Knighton RW, Huang XR. Effect of corneal polarization axis on assessment of retinal nerve fiber layer thickness by scanning laser polarimetry. Am J Ophthalmol 2000;129:715-722.
29) Tjon Fo Sang MJ, Lemji HG. Sensitivity and specificity of nerve fiber layer measurement in glaucoma as determined with scanning laser polarimetry. Am J Ophthalmol 1997;123:62-69.
30) Schuman JS, Hee MR, Puliafito CA, et al. Quantification of nerve fiber layer thickness in normal and glaucomatous eyes using optical coherence tomography. A pilot study. Arch Ophthalmol 1995;113:586-596.

31) Carpineto P, Ciancaglini M, Zuppardi E, et al. Reliability of nerve fiber layer thickness measurement using OCT in normal and glaucomatous patients. Ophthalmology 2003;110:190-195.
32) Parisi V, Manni G, Centofanti M, et a. Correlation between optical coherence tomography, pattern electroretinogram, and visual evoked potentials in open-angle glaucoma patients. Ophthalmology 2001;108:905-912.
33) Zeimer R, Asrani S, Zou S, Quigley H, Jampel H. Quantitative detection of glaucomatous damage at the posterior pole by retinal thickness mapping. Ophthalmology 1998;105:224-231.
34) Brusini P, Tosoni C, Miani F. Retinal thickness measurements in chronic glaucoma and ocular hypertension. Perimetry Update 2000/2001, Kugler Publ, The Hague, The Netherlands 2001;29-34.
35) Spaeth GL, Katz LJ, Terebuth AK. Managing glaucoma on the basis of tissue damage: a therapeutic approach based largely on the appearance of the optic disc. In: Krieglestein GK (eds). Glaucoma Update V. Kaden, 1995.
36) Fazio P, Krupin T, Feitl ME, Werner EB, Carrè DA. Optic disc topography in patients with low-tension and primary open-angle glaucoma. Arch Ophthalmol 1990;108:705-708.
37) Miller KM, Quigley HA. Comparison of optic disc features in low-tension and typical open-angle glaucoma. Ophthal Surg 1987;18:882-889.
38) Caprioli J, Spaeth GL. Comparison of the optic nerve head in high- and low-tension glaucoma. Arch Ophthalmol 1985;103:1145-1149.
39) Bayer A, Hararymowycz P, Henderer JD, Steissmann WG, Spaeth G. Validity of a new disk grading scale for etimating glaucomatous damage: consideration with visual field damage. Am J Ophthalmol 2002;133:758-763.
40) Goji T. The optic nerve head in normal-tension glaucoma. Curr Opin Ophthalmol 2000;11:116-120.
41) Iester M, Mikelberg FS. Optic nerve head morphologic characteristics in high-tension and normal-tension glaucoma. Arch Ophthalmol 1999;117:1010-1013.
42) Chauhan BC, McCormick TA, Nicolela MT, LeBlanc RP. Optic disc and visual field changes in a prospective \ longitudinal study of patients with glaucoma. Comparison of scanning laser tomography with conventional perimetry and optic disc photography. Arch Ophthalmol 2001;119:1492-1499.
43) Kamal DS, Garway-Heath DF, Hitchings RA, Fitzke FW. Use of sequential Heidelberg retina tomograph images to identify changes at the optic disc in ocular hypertensive patients at risk of developing glaucoma. Br J Ophthalmol 2000;84:993-998.
44) Spaeth GL. Development of glaucomatous changes of the optic nerve. In: Varma R, Spaeth GL, Parker KW (eds). The optic nerve in glaucoma. Philadelphia, JB Lippincott, 1993.
45) Jonas JB. Biomorphometric des Nervus optikus. Stuttgart, Enke-Verlag, 1990.
46) Tuulonen A, Airaksinen PJ. Initial Galucomatous optic disk and retinal nerve fiber layer abnormalities and their progression. Am J Ophthalmol 1991;111:485-490.
47) Quigley HA. II. Changes in the appearance of the optic disk. Surv Ophthalmol 1985;30:117-126.
48) Henderer JD, Liu C, Kesen M, Altangered U, Bayer A, Steinmann WC, Spaeth GL. Reliability of the disk damage likelihood scale. Am J Ophthalmol 2003;15:44-48.

1.4 - VISUAL FIELD

The field of vision is defined as the area that is perceived when both eyes are open. Clinically, each eye is assessed independently. Please see FC II, III, IV.

There are two main methods of testing the visual field (VF):

A) *Kinetic perimetry*: a stimulus is moved from a nonseeing area of the visual field to a seeing area along a set meridian. The procedure is repeated with the same stimulus along other meridians, usually spaced every 15°. The luminance and size of the target is changed in order to plot areas of different light sensitivity.
B) *Static perimetry*: the size and location of the test target remain constant. The retinal sensitivity or threshold at a specific location is determined by varying the brightness of the test target. The shape of the hill of vision is defined by repeating the threshold measurement at various locations in the field of vision.

In this chapter we refer mainly to Humphrey and Octopus perimeters, which are the most popular in Europe; several other brands offer similar examination capabilities.

1.4.1 - APOSTILBS & DECIBELS

In perimetry the luminance of the test target is measured in Apostilbs (asb).
1 asb = 0.3183 candela/m2 = 0.1 millilambert
The decibel scale is a relative scale created by the manufacturers of automated perimeters to measure the sensitivity each tested point of the hill of vision. It is an inverted logarithmic scale. Zero decibels is set as the brightest stimulus

Apostilbs	Humphrey Decibels	Octopus Decibels
0.1	50	40
1	40	30
1000	10	0
10000	0	-

1 bel = 1 log Unit = tenfold change in intensity
1 decibel = 0.1 log Unit
Decibel = dB

that each perimeter can produce. The decibel scale is not standardised because the maximal luminance of the stimulus varies between instruments.
It is important to note that:
1) "0" dB do not correspond to the same stimulus luminance for Humphrey and Octopus
2) "0" dB does not mean a blind area but rather an area where the sensitivity of the retina to the stimulus is below the maximum brightness for a given perimeter.

1.4.2 - STATIC VISUAL FIELD EXAM

1.4.2.1 - Reference tests for glaucoma

1.4.2.1.1 - Conventional techniques

Humphrey Perimeter, programs 24-2 or 30-2, or Octopus 32 measure the retinal sensitivity at 54 or 76 points in the

central 24 or 30 central degrees respectively. Testing points are aligned 3° off the vertical and horizontal meridians in order to facilitate detection of "nasal steps" field defects.
Octopus Program G1 measures the retinal sensitivity at 73 points. 59 points are in the central 26 degrees (phase 1 and 2) at full threshold; 14 points are in the periphery, between 30 and 60 degrees (phase 3), and are tested at suprathreshold levels.

SITA Standard and Fast for Humphrey and TOP for Octopus
Offers the advantage of a short test time.
Available data are promising but need to be confirmed before this technique is generally applied[1].
Exams performed with the same instrument but with different strategies should not be used to assess progression.

1.4.2.1.2 - Non conventional techniques

SWAP (Short Wavelength Automated Perimetry) is based on the theory that the yellow light of the background can reduce the sensitivity of some photoreceptors and leave active the blue cones that carry the stimulus using "Parvo" ganglion cells. It is greatly affected by lens density.

FDT (Frequency doubling technology) is based on the theory that "My "ganglion cells are the first to be involved in glaucoma and that using low spatial and high temporal frequency stimuli it is possible to detect the loss of these cells. Motion and Flicker perimetry have been applied in clinical research; further developments are pending.

HRP (High Pass Resolution Perimetry) is based on the theory that "Parvo" ganglion cells can be detected particularly well by high spatial and low temporal stimuli. This technology not been widely disseminated.

Available data are promising especially for early detection of functional damage. The role of these techniques in the routine management is yet to be defined[2-10].

1.4.3 - THE EVALUATION OF PERIMETRY EXAMINATION

Possible sources of errors:

- Name: if mistyped the patient can be easily misdiagnosed, and the automated analysis of progression during the follow-up is impossible.
- Date of the exam
- Birthdate: if mistyped patient identification is not possible, and the analysis may be incorrect, since threshold testing takes into account age in the normative database. After the age of 20 there is a loss of differential light sensitivity of 0.6 dB per decade, which is more pronounced in the peripheral visual field. If a false lower age is entered, the normal field is evaluated as a field with pathologically low sensitivity; if false higher age is entered, even pathological visual fields can be evaluated as normal.
- Refraction: the test should be done using near vision correction after the age of 40 or in aphakes and pseudophakes. Astigmatism of more than 1 diopter can produce a refractive temporal peripheral scotoma. If the correcting lens is not centered, a peripheral scotoma can be observed. Aphakic spectacle correction causes up to 50% of constriction of the visual field (called annular scotoma). An anterior chamber intraocular lens can cause a slight constriction of the visual field.
- Pupil size: ideally 3.5 to 4 mm. Very small and very dilated pupils cause low or high sensitivity, respectively, which may be misleading both as regards diagnosis and the evaluation of progression. If the size of the pupil is outside the normal range (2 to 4 mm diameter) when the visual field is tested, the influence of the pupil-size must be considered.
- Strategy / method / program: Differences between the algorithms used for sensitivity testing and processing cause differences in the indices shown in the report. This must be considered when the visual field is evaluated. In general, shorter programs (Humphrey, SITA, Octopus TOP Dynamic test) show better sensitivity (i.e. smaller MD) than conventional, longer programs (e.g. Humphrey full threshold test or OCTOPUS normal strategy).
- Duration of the test: approximately 15 minutes per eye. Poor reliability should be suspected if the test time is too long. In these cases a shorter test should be considered. Fatigue can be responsible for false visual field defects

- Number of visual fields previously performed: a learning effect is demonstrable with automated perimetry[11]. This should be taken into account when evaluating the initial fields and comparing results with later tests.
- Eyelid position: ptosis or blepharochalasis can result in a false superior scotoma.
- Reliability indices:

  * fixation losses: if fixation losses exceed 20-30% and the blind spot was correctly plotted at the start of the test, reliability should be questioned.

  * false positive: if the patient responds without a stimulus being presented, this is considered a false positive. False positive answers can make the visual field look better than it actually is. If false positives exceed 20%, reliability should be questioned.

  * false negative: a test point of known light sensitivity is rechecked with a brighter stimulus. If there is no response a false negative response is recorded. False negatives are a sign of poor reliability, and also of advanced glaucomatous damage and can make the visual field look worse than it actually is. If false negatives exceed 20%, reliability should be questioned.

Duties of the perimeter "user"

Positioning the patient: to help the subject to a convenient position for the test, and to correct the anatomical features (e.g. overhanging eyelids) which may potentially influence the test
Patient instruction/training: to inform and to train the subject regarding the test (e.g. how to respond, how to rest in case of fatigue etc.)
Refractive correction: to correct ametropia for near in a technically correct manner
Documentation: to evaluate and document any other test characteristics (e.g. "I corrected the ptosis of the left eye" or "the subject was very nervous during the test") in order to assist the decision made by the treating ophthalmologist.

PRACTICALITIES ON VISUAL FIELD EXAMINATION

* Most patients become more proficient after their first examination. This effect shows as an improvement in the test and is called "learning effect". The first tests in a perimetrically naive subject should be considered with caution or discarded.

* To be clinically significant, a visual field defect must be real. To be real, it must be confirmed on repeated exams.

* Media opacity and miotic pupils worsen the MD through a generalized depression of sensitivity.

* Disc features must match the visual field defects.

* Rule out other ocular causes of visual field defects i.e. retinochoroidal lesions.

Assessing the test results

Grey scale: This allows a quick overview but should not be used for quantitative evaluation.
Decibel values: This gives the differential light sensitivity of each tested point. Some locations are tested twice.
Ideally the sensitivity of each point should be compared in successive visual fields (Peridata, Glaucoma Change Probability or Progressor programs).
Total deviation: The difference between the differential light sensitivity values measured in the patient and normal dB values for age and eccentricity.

Global indices[12]:

• MD (mean defect or mean deviation): this is the mean difference between the normal sensitivity (corrected for age) and the retinal sensitivity for the subject (calculated from all the points tested). MD increases with the following: media opacities, diffuse loss or severe localised loss.

A retinal sensitivity value worse than normal is indicated by a negative symbol in Humphrey perimeters (mean deviation) and a positive symbol in Octopus perimeters (mean defect).

• PSD or LV (pattern standard deviation or loss variance): this is the standard deviation or variance of the deviations and is thus a measure of the degree to which the shape of a patient's field differs from a normal, age-corrected, reference field. Thus the PSD or LV indicate the extent of focal loss in the visual field. The PSD or LV can be normal in cases where there is diffuse loss and they are not good indices for the follow up of advanced glaucoma.

• SF (short term fluctuation): this indicates variability during a test at points that are tested twice; it is generally higher in fields with glaucomatous damage. SF is thus an index of the patient's consistency during the test period.

• CPSD or CLV (corrected pattern standard deviation or corrected loss variance): this indicates the extent of focal loss in the visual field, taking short term fluctuation into account.

• Probability indices : abnormal global indices are presented with a probability denoted p < 'x'%, indicating that there is 'an 'x'% chance that this index is in reality normal.

Bebié Curve or Cumulative Defect Curve (Octopus, Peridata): the 59 points tested at full threshold (in the G1 program) are ranked from the highest to the lowest sensitivity after age correction. A curve is obtained where the points on the left represent the better points in the visual field and those on the right the worse points[13].

When the sensitivity loss is diffuse most of or all the curve is not within the 95% prediction interval of the normal population curve.

When the sensitivity loss is localised, and the sensitivity at some points is normal and at others abnormal, the patient's curve is within normal limits on the left and drops down sharply to the right.

Glaucoma hemifield test: this compares each of 5 groups of test points tested in a hemifield with the corresponding group in the opposite hemifield. It is reported as abnormal, borderline or normal[14].

DIAGNOSTIC CRITERIA FOR GLAUCOMATOUS VISUAL FIELD LOSS

(in the absence of retinal or neurological disease affecting visual field)

Visual field loss is considered significant when:

a) abnormal Glaucoma Hemifield Test, confirmed on two consecutive tests[15], or

b) 3 abnormal points confirmed on two consecutive tests, with p < 5% probability of being normal,
one of which should have p < 1%, all being not contiguous with the blind spot,

c) CPSD < 5% if the visual field is otherwise normal, confirmed on two consecutive tests.

Any defect or suspected defect must be confirmed by repeated testing.

1.4.4 - GRADING SYSTEMS[16]

Scoring based on defect extent and on proximity of the defect to fixation point

Hodapp and co-workers proposed a classification in three stages considering MD value, number of depressed test sites on the pattern deviation map and the presence of defect sites within the central 5°. This type of scoring needs an accurate analysis of visual field which is useful but time-consuming[17]. It emphasizes the closeness of defective points to the fixation.

Grading based on kinetic perimetry

Aulhorn and Kermeyer 's classification based on kinetic and profile static perimetry patterns includes five stages of increasing severity, according to visual field defects extension and morphology[18].

The advantage of this classification is that it is simple and immediately understandable; disadvantages are that it is quite subjective and not very reproducible, because it is largely based on personal experience in evaluating the visual field. Manual perimetry is used less and less nowadays.

Grading based on number and depth of defect points

The Advanced Glaucoma Intervention Study (AGIS) investigators proposed a classification where the VF defect score is based on the number and depth of clusters of adjacent depressed test sites in the upper and lower hemifields and in the nasal area of the total deviation print out (Statpac 2 analysis)[19]. The score ranges from 0 (no defect) to 20 (all test sites deeply depressed). This scoring system is accurate. For routine use however it might be too elaborate. Langerhorst using scoperimeter (experimental perimeter) data suggested a classification in five stages[20]. This type of classification can be adapted to standard full threshold programs, like Humphrey 30-2 or Octopus G1.

Esterman grids

Esterman proposed a visual field defect quantification system, using a 100 sector grid, denser in the central and inferior area of the visual field[21]. This grid must be superimposed on VF, in order to obtain a score showing VF functional state. Drawback of this method is that it only applies to supraliminal strategies and is not useful in glaucoma staging.
This classification was modified for threshold strategies in order to obtain more information on functional status.

Classification based on perimetric indices

Perimetric indices were proposed first by Flammer for Octopus perimeters and are available also for the majority of other instruments[9]. The most revelant indices are mean sensitivity (MS), mean deviation or mean defect (MD), loss variance (LV), pattern standard deviation (PSD), short-term fluctuation (SF), corrected loss variance (CLV), corrected pattern standard deviation (CPSD). Various indices can be used to stage glaucomatous damage.
It was noted that CLV was elevated in the first phases of glaucoma and the elevated level of CLV did not vary with increasing field loss as indicated by MD[24]. A classification system for defining stages of glaucoma was proposed utilizing CLV and MD as a combined index. CLV was shown to be sensitive to early stages of glaucoma damage, subsequently becoming stable.
MD was shown to be sensitive to progression of field loss, but not useful for early detection. It may be advantageous to combine these two field indices in order to achieve a more comprehensive picture of field loss in glaucoma.
Brusini proposed a staging system using MD, CLV and CPSD[25,26]. This method requires the use of specific charts.
It is very rapid and practical for clinical use, and it is gaining popularity. It allows to grade the severity and the type of the defect, but is not specific for glaucoma.

Staging based on Statpac box-plot

Shin and co-workers developed a system for classification of glaucomatous VF defects by means of numerical values[27]. The visual fields were represented by Humphrey Box-plots and were classified by the minimum, the lower limit of the box and the median.
The VF defect can be classified into five major stages and five minor groups. This method objectively represents the extent of the VF defects, but does not indicate the type.

Glaucoma change probability analysis (Statpac 2 - Humphrey)

This program allows selection of two early visual field tests as baseline. Subsequent visual fields are directly compared to this baseline. Significant change from baseline in the measured threshold at any location is determined by comparison with reference database of visual fields from stable glaucoma subjects. This probability analysis has been shown to correlate well with routine clinical evaluation of progression of visual field changes[28].

Progressor (Pointwise linear regression analysis)

All the luminance sensitivity measurements are analyzed by linear regression that generates a slope at each location with a positive or negative sign and a p value[29,30].
An excellent test for longitudinal follow-up. It requires proprietary software.

<u>Please note: none of the grading systems is specific for glaucoma.</u>

HODAPP CLASSIFICATION[31]

EARLY GLAUCOMATOUS LOSS

a) MD > - 6 dB

b) Fewer than 18 points depressed below the 5% probability level and fewer than 10 points below the p < 1% level

c) No point in the central 5 degrees with a sensitivity of less than 15 dB

MODERATE GLAUCOMATOUS LOSS

a) -6 > MD > -12 dB

b) Fewer than 37 points depressed below the 5% probability level and fewer than 20 points below the p < 1% level

c) No absolute deficit (0 dB) in the 5 central degrees

d) Only one hemifield with sensitivity of < 15 dB in the 5 central degrees

ADVANCED GLAUCOMATOUS LOSS

a) MD < -12 dB

b) More than 37 points depressed below the 5% probability level or more than 20 points below the p < 1% level

c) Absolute deficit (0 dB) in the 5 central degrees

d) Sensitivity < 15 dB in the 5 central degrees in both hemifields

1.4.5 - WORSENING OF THE VISUAL FIELD

Looking for visual field progression is the most important part of clinical management in chronic glaucoma because this is the outcome that affects the patients quality of life. Changes in the visual field will make the Physician consider a change in clinical management The identification of visual field progression requires a series of fields, usually more than three, and often 5 or 6. Diagnosing visual field progession on a shorter visual field series is risky, because of the inherent variability in patient responses. The exception would be a dramatic change that was associated with corresponding symptoms suggesting visual loss and confirmed by unquestionable changes in ONH/RNFL. In many instances of such sudden change, the cause will not be glaucoma, but either vascular in origin, or due to changes in the visual pathways.

Recent Treatment/No Treatment trials (see Introduction) have shown that glaucomatous field progression is usually slow, and that it will rarely be detected within one year of followup, even with a strict test/retest regime. In clinical practice there will be an individual approach, with stricter follow up being indicated in cases with advanced disease or with VF defects close to fixation. A practical scheme is to perform 2-3 tests that 'train' the patient, and provide mean values for a baseline, and then to repeat testing twice a year. A clinical routine that involves less frequent testing will reduce the chances of identifying change.

Reduced sensitivity in a cluster of test points on the same hemifield, and outside the periphery by >=5db, or a single test point by > 10 db needs confirmation. This confirmation needs to be obtained on 2 subsequent field tests before deemed a permanent change.

As an example, when using the Glaucoma Change Probability Maps in the Humphrey perimeter, at least three points flagged as significantly progressing that occur in the same location in three consecutive examinations can be used to define 'confirmed' glaucomatous field progression; the same pattern occurring in two consecutive fields can be used to denote 'tentative' field progression.

SUMMARY OF SUGGESTED CRITERIA FOR VISUAL FIELD DEFECT PROGRESSION*

For a new defect in a previous normal area

- A cluster of three or more non-edge points, each of which declines ≥ 5 dB compared to baseline on two consecutive fields.

or

- A single non-edge point that declines ≥10 dB compared to baseline on two consecutive fields.

or

- A cluster of three or more non-edge points, each of which declines at a $p < 5\%$ level compared to baseline on two consecutive fields.

For deepening of a preexisting defect

- A cluster of three non-edge points, each of which declines ≥ 10 dB compared to baseline on two consecutive fields. The confirming points may differ if they are part of a contiguous cluster.

or

- A cluster of three non-edge points or three points that are part of the same scotoma, each of which worsens at least 5 dB and is depressed compared to baseline at a $p < 5\%$ level on two consecutive fields. The confirming points may differ if they are part of a contiguous cluster or are separated by points not in the data base.

For expansion of preexisting scotoma into contiguous points

- At least two previously normal points within the central 15° or three additional previously normal points outside at the central 15°, each of which declines ≥ 10 dB each on two consecutive fields.

or

- At least two previously normal points within the central 15° or three previously normal points outside 15°, each of which is depressed at a $p < 5\%$ level compared to baseline on two consecutive fields.

For generalized depression

- A decline in the mean deviation that is significant at the $p < 1\%$ level and is not explained by media opacity or pupil size.

or

- A CPSD that shows an obvious trend based on the last five consecutive fields.

or

- A decline of ≥ 3 dB at all points on two consecutive fields that is not explained by media opacity or pupil size.

PROGRESSION MUST BE CONFIRMED

* Modified from Hodapp et Al[31]

References

1) Bengtsson B, Heijl A, Olsson J. Evaluation of a new hreshold visual field strategy, SITA, in normal subjects. Acta Ophthalmol Scand 1998;76:165-169.
2) Sample PA, Taylor JDN, Martinez GA, Lusky M, Weinreb RN. Short-wave lenght colour visual field in glaucoma suspect at risk. Am J Ophthalmol 1993;115:225-233.
3) Felius J, De Long LAS, Van de Berg TP, Greve EL. Functional characteristics of blue on yellow perimetric thres holds in glaucoma. Invest Ophthalmol Vis Sci 1995;36:1665-1674.
4) Frisèn L. High-Pass Resolution perimetry. Recent development. In Heijl A (eds). Perimetry update 1988/89. Berkeley-Milano, Kugler-Ghedini 1989,369-375.
5) Iester M, Alteri M, Vittone P, Calabria G, ZingirianM, Traverso CE. Detection of glaucomatous visual field defect by non-conventional perimetry. Am J Opthalmol 2003;135:35-39.
6) Johnson CA, Samuel SJ. Screening for glaucomatous visual field loss with frequency doubling perimetry. Invest OphthalmolVis Sci 1997;38:413-425.
7) Iester M, Mermoud A, Schnyder C. Frequency Doubling Technique in subject with ocular hypertension and glaucoma. Correlation with Octopus Perimeter Indices. Opthalmology 2001;107:228-294.
8) Wall M, Ketoff KM. Random dot motion perimetry in patients with glaucoma and in normal subjects. Am J Ophthalmol 1995;120:587-596.
9) Lachenmayer BJ, Drance SM, Chauhan BC, House PH, Lalani S. Diffuse and localized glaucomatous field loss in light-sense flicker and resolution perimetry. Graefe's Arch Clin Exp Ophthalmol 1991;229:246-251.
10) Brusini P, Tosoni C. Staging of functional damage in glaucoma using frequency doubling techology. J Glaucoma (in press).
11) Heijl A, Bengtsson B. The effect of perimetric experience in patients with glaucoma. Arch Ophthalmol 1996;114:19-22.
12) Flammer J. The concept of visual field indices. Graefe's Arch Clin Exp Ophthalmol 1986;224:389-392.
13) Bebie H, Flammer J, Bebie Th. The cumulative defect curve: separation of local and diffuse components of visual field damage. Graefe's Arch Clin Exp Ophthalmol 1989;227:9-12.
14) Aasman P, Heijl A. Evaluation of methods for automated hemifield analysis in perimetry. Arch Ophthalmol 1992;110:812-819.
15) Katz J, Quigley HA, Sommer A. Detection of incident field loss using the glaucoma hemifield test. Ophthalmology 1996;103:657-663.
16) Brusini P. Stadiazione del difetto perimetrico nel glaucoma. Oftalmografia, 2, Ed. Innovation-News-Communication, Roma, 1996.
17) Hodapp E, Parrish IIRK, Anderson DR. Clinical decision in glaucoma. St Louis, CV Mosby Comp 1993;52-61.
18) Aulhorm E, Karmeyer H. Frequency distribution in early glaucomatous visual field defects. Doc Ophthalmol Proc Series 1977;14:75-83.
19) The Advanced Glaucoma Intervention Study Investigators: Advanced Glaucoma Intervention Study. Visual field test scoring and reliability. Ophthalmology 1994;101:1445-1455.
20) Langerhorst CT, van den Berg TJTP, Greve EL. Fluctuation and general health in automated perimetry in glaucoma. In Heijl A (eds). Perimetry update 1988/89. Berkeley-Milano, Kugler-Ghedini 1989,159-164.
21) Estermann B. Grid for scoring visual fields. II Perimeter. Arch Ophthalmol 1968;79:400-406.
22) Del Vecchio GC, Brombin A, Cavallini GM, Bussolari L. Metodo di calcolo per l'assegnazione di un punteggio al campo visivo computerizzato di soglia. Minerva Oftalmol 1998;40:95-101.
23) Gandolfo E, Zingirian M, Capris P. A new proposal for classification and quantification of visual field disability. In: Mills RP, Heijl A (eds). Perimetry update 1990-91, Amsterdam, New York, Kugler publ, 1991;545-549.
24) Gollamudi S, Liao P, Hirsch J. Evaluation of corrected loss variance as a visual field index. Corrected loss variance in conjunction with mean defect may identify stages of glaucoma. Ophthalmologica 1988;197:144-150.
25) Brusini P. Clinical use of a new method for visual field damage classification in glaucoma. Eur J Ophthalmol 1996;6:402-407.
26) Kocak I, Zulauf M, Hendrickson P, Stumpfig D. Evaluation of the Brusini glaucoma staging system for follow-up in glaucoma. Eur J Ophthalmol 1997;7:345-350.
27) Shin YS, Suzumura H, Furuno, Harasawa K, Endo N, Matsuo H. Classification of glaucomatous visual field defect using the Humphrey field analizer Box-plots. In: Mills RP, Heel A (eds) Perimetry Update 1990-91, Amsterdam, New York, Kugler, 1991;235-243.

28) Mc Naught AI, Crabb DP, Fitzke FW, Hitchings RA. Visual field progression: comparison of Humphrey Statpac 2 and point-wise linear regression analysis. Graefe's Arch Clin Exp Ophthalmol 1996;243:411-418.
29) Birch MK, Wishart PK, O'Donnell NP. Determining progressive visual field loss in serial Humphrey visual fields. Ophthalmology 1995;102:1227-1235.
30) Fitzke FW, Hitchings RA, Poinoosawmy D, Mc Naught AI, Crabb DP. Analysis of visual field progression in glaucoma. Br J Ophthalmol 1996;80:40-46.
31) Hodapp E, Parrish IIRK, Anderson DR. Clinical decisions in glaucoma. St Louis, The CV Mosby, 1993;84-126.

1.5 - BLOOD FLOW

1.5.1 - VASCULAR FACTORS AND GLAUCOMA

Factors involved in the aetiology and progression of glaucomatous optic neuropathy are not only pressure dependent and are also related to the vascular supply of the optic nerve head.

Many observations indicate the need to study the relationship between blood flow and glaucoma:
- existence of normal tension glaucoma (NTG)[1-4]
- presence of disc haemorrhages in glaucoma patients
- higher prevalence of retinal vein occlusion in glaucoma patients
- association of NTG and migraine, Raynaud's phenomenon, vasospasm[5,6,7]
- association of NTG and systemic hypotension and excessive number of nocturnal "dips" in diastolic blood pressure[8,9]
- association of glaucoma and abnormal blood coagulability profile[10,11]
- association of NTG and silent myocadial ischaemia[9]
- association of glaucoma (NTG) and cerebral infarcts[12,16]
- association of NTG and an history of hypotensive shock or episode of severe blood loss.[5]

1.5.2 - MEASUREMENTS METHODS OF OCULAR BLOOD FLOW

Many methods have been used to calculate ocular blood flow: fluorescein angiography[14,15], scanning laser ophthalmoscope[16], videoangiography[17,18], laser Doppler velocimetry[19,20], laser speckle phenomenon, blue field entoptic phenomenon[21], pulsatile ocular blood flow[22], colour Doppler imaging[23,24], oculodynamography[25-27]. For technical reasons, wide interindividual variations can occur with problems related to posture, as well as technician experience, patient cooperation. Multiple measurements are therefore required. More importantly in glaucoma, it is relevant to measure the blood supply to the retrolaminar portion of the optic nerve head, i.e. small vessels which are difficult to visualise and have wide anatomic variability.
The number of methods used illustrate the difficulty of measurements of ocular blood flow relative to the blood supply of the optic nerve head, size of of vessels, individual variations, reproducibility of measurements techniques.

At the present time the clinical role of blood flow measurements in glaucoma management (and the relevance of changes noted with drug treatments) are unclear and these techniques remain research tools.

However clinical vascular risk factors should be taken into account in glaucoma management especially when the IOP is low (over 24 hours and with normal CCT) and visual fields show severe and progressive alteration[28].

1.6 - AXIAL LENGTH MEASUREMENTS

For follow-up of congenital glaucoma axial length measurement is a useful tool, especially to correlate with IOP findings, refraction and corneal diameter[29,30].

References

1) Pillunat LE, Stodtmeister R, Marquardt R, Mattern A. Ocular perfusion pressures in different types of glaucoma. Int Ophthalmol 1989;13:37-42.
2) Nicolela MT, Walman BE, Buckley AR, Drance SM. Ocular hypertension and primary open-angle glaucoma: a comparative study of their retrobulbar blood flow velocity. J Glaucoma 1996;5:308-310.
3) Nicolela MT, Hnik P, Drance SM. Scanning laser Doppler flowmeter study of retinal and optic disk blood flow in glaucomatous patients. Am J Ophthalmol 1996;122:775-783.
4) O'Brien C, Saxton V, Crick RP, Meire H. Doppler carotid artery studies in asymmetric glaucoma. Eye 1992;6:273-276.
5) Drance SM. Some factors in the production of low tension glaucoma. Br J Ophthalmol 1972 56(3):229-242.
6) Fechtner R, Weinreb R. Mechanisms of optic nerve damage in primary open-angle glaucoma. Surv Ophthalmol 1994;39:23-42.
7) Phelps CD, CorbettJJ. Migraine and low tension glaucoma. A case control sudy. Invest Ophthalmol Vis Sci. 1985;26:1105-1108.
8) Hayreh SS, Zimmerman, Podhajsky P, Alward WLM. Nocturnal arterial hypotension and its role in optic nerve head and ocular ischemic disorders. Am J Ophthalmol 1994,117:603-624.
9) Kaiser HJ, Flammer J, Graf T, Stumpfig D. Systemic blood pressure in glaucoma patients. Graefes Arch Clin Exp Ophthalmol 1993;231:677-680.
10) Hamard P, Hamard H, Dufaux J et al. Optic nerve head blood flow using a laser doppler velocimeter and haemorheology in primary open-angle glaucoma and normal pressure glaucoma. Br J Ophthalmol 1994;78:449-453.
11) Mary A, Serre I, Brun J-F, et al. Erythrocyte deformability measurements in patients with glaucoma. J Glaucoma 1993;2:155-157.
12) Ong K, Farinelli A, Bilson F et al. Comparative study of brain magnetic resonance imaging findings in patients with low tension glaucoma and control subjects. Ophthalmology 1995;102:1632-1638.
13) Stroman, G Golnik, K., Hund, P. Magnetic Resonance Imaging in patients with Unexplained Optic Neuropathy. Arch Ophthalmol 1995;113:1041-1044.
14) Cantor LB, Harris A, Wolf S, Sponsel W, Arend O. Measurement of superficial optic nerve head capillary blood velocities by scanning laser fluorescein angiography. J Glaucoma 1994;3:S61-S64.
15) Koyama T, Matsuo N, Shimizu K, Mihara M, Tsuchida Y et al. Retinal circulation times in quantitative fluorescein angiography. Graefes Arch Clin Exp Ophthalmol 1990;228(5):442-446.
16) Ulrich WD, Ulrich C, Walter G. Ocular perfusion pressure and ocullo-oscillo-dynamography. In: Ocular Blood Flow in Glaucoma. Lambrou GN, Greve EL, Kugler ang Ghedini, ed 1989;101-115.
17) Tanaka Y. Color-fluorescein relationship in glaucomatous optic damage. Jpn J Ophthalmol 1995;39:180-186.
18) Laatikainen L. Fluorescein angiographic studies of the peripapillary and perilimbal regions in simple, capsular and low-tension glaucoma. Acta Ophthalmol Suppl 1971;111:3-83.
19) Iester M, Altieri M, Michelson G, Vittone P, Calabria G, Traverso CE. Intraobserver riproducibility of a two dimensional mapping of the optic nerve head perfusion. J Glaucoma 2002;11:488-492.
20) Michelson G, Schmauss B. Two dimensional mapping of the perfusion of the retina and optic nerve head. Br J Ophthalmol 1995;79:1126-1132.
21) Riva CE, Petrig B. Blue field entoptic phenomenon and blood velocity in the retinal capillaries. J Op Soc Am 1980;70:1234-1238.
22) Butt Z, O'Brien C. Reproducibility of pulsatile ocular blood flow measurements. J Glaucoma 1995;4:214-218.
23) Williamson TH, Harris A. Color Doppler ultrasound imaging of the eye and orbit. Surv Ophthalmol 1996;40:255-267.
24) Lachkar Y, Migdal C Danjil S. Effect of Brimonidine tartrate on ocular hemodynamic measurements. Arch Ophthalmol 1998;116:1591-1594.
25) Jonas JB. Ophthalmodynamometry in eyes with dilated episcleral veins. J Glaucoma 2003;12:282-287.
26) Jonas JB, Niessen A. Ophthalmodynamometric diagnosis of unilateral ischemic ophthalmopathy. Am J Ophthalmol 2002;134:911-912.
27) Jonas JB. Reproducibility of ophthalmodynamometric measurements of central retinal artery and vein collapse pressure. Br J Opthalmol 2003;87:577-579.

28) Flammer J, Orgul S, Costa VP, Orzalesi N, Krieglstein GK, Serra LM, Renard JP, Stefansson E. The impact of ocular blood flow in glaucoma. Prog Retin Eye Res 2002;21:359-393
29) Reibaldi A, Biometric ultrasound in the diagnosis and follow-up of congenital glaucoma. Ann Ophthalmol 1982;14:707-708.
30) Sampaolesi R. Corneal diameter and axial length in congenital glaucoma. Can J Ophthalmol 1988;2:42-44.

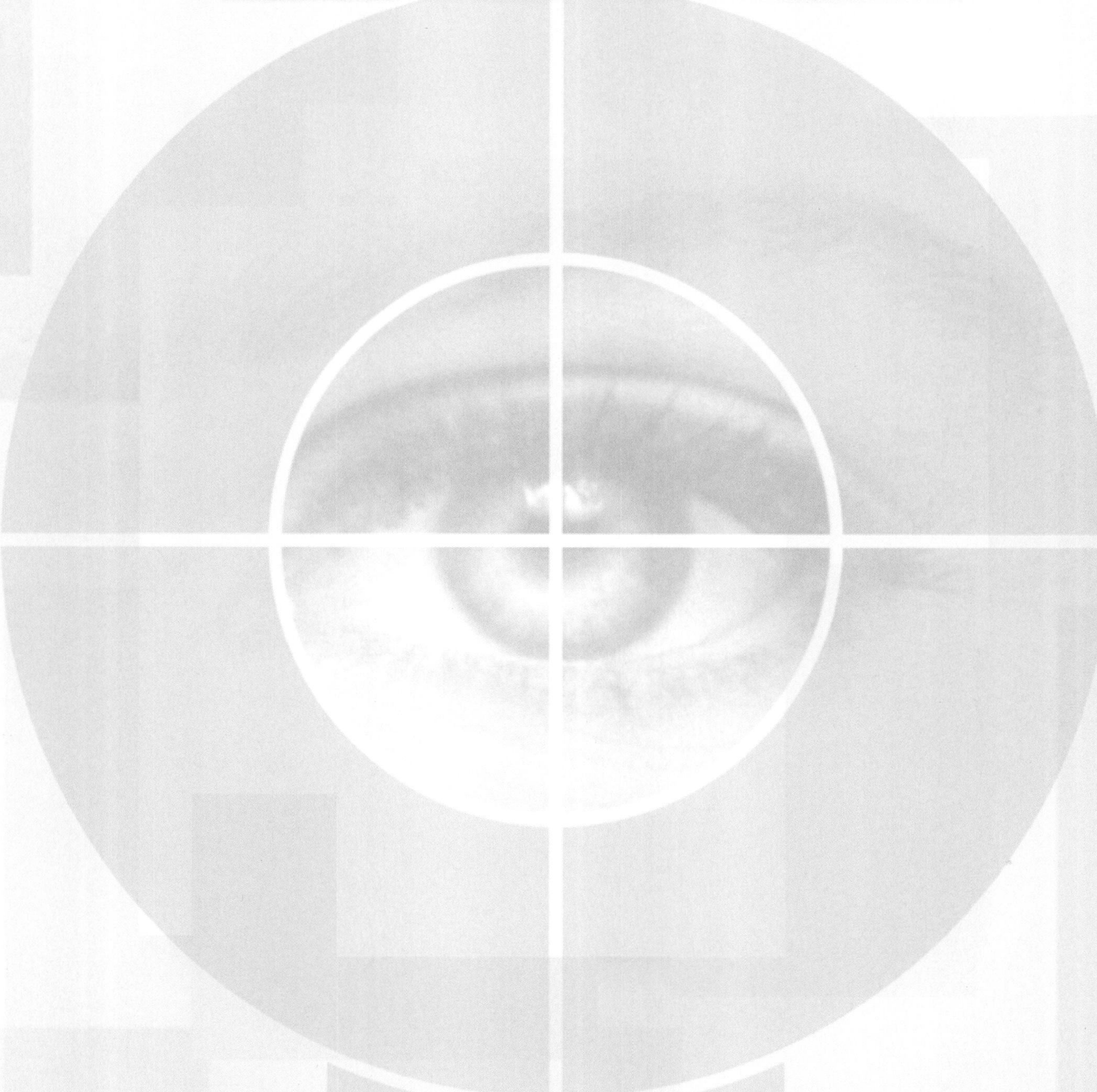

CHAPTER 2

CLASSIFICATION AND TERMINOLOGY

All forms of glaucoma should be classified into primary and secondary forms based on:

* Anterior chamber angle at gonioscopy
* Optic nerve head findings
* Visual field defects

* Major risk factors:
Intra-ocular pressure (IOP)
Age
Vascular risk factors:
- local
- systemic
Low diastolic perfusion pressure
Race (particularly Afro-Caribbean)

* Associated conditions:
Ocular
Extraocular

Additional Useful Clinical Data

- Blood pressure
- Heart rate
- Blood sugar
- Blood lipids
- Migraine
- Cold hands, Raynaud's
- Neurological diseases
- Thyroid disease
- History of blood loss
- History of kidney disease
- Smoking habits
- Drinking habits
- Family history of visual loss
- Family history of glaucoma

The role of diabetes mellitus as a risk factor for the development of POAG is controversial.

2.1 - PRIMARY CONGENITAL FORMS

2.1.1 - PRIMARY CONGENITAL GLAUCOMA

Etiology: Angle dysgenesis
Pathomechanism: Decreased aqueous outflow
Features:

- Onset: from birth to second year of life
- Heredity: usually sporadic, up to 10% recessive inheritance with variable penetrance
- Gender: more common in males (65%)
- Specific chromosomal abnormalities have been identified at 1p36 and 2q21
- Signs and symptoms:
  - Photophobia, tearing, blepharospasm, eye rubbing
  - IOP in general anesthesia: insufficient alone to confirm the diagnosis unless extremely elevated since general anesthesia may lower the IOP
  - Corneal diameter > 11 mm (buphthalmos)
  - Corneal edema (+/- ruptures of Descemet's Membrane.)
  - Optic nerve head: pressure distension/uniform cup enlargement (CDR >0.3)
  - Gonioscopy: open-angle
    - poorly differentiated structures
    - trabeculodysgenesis (including 'Barkan's membrane')
    - anterior insertion of the iris

2.1.2 - PRIMARY INFANTILE GLAUCOMA / Late-Onset Primary Congenital Glaucoma

Etiology: Angle dysgenesis
Pathomechanism: Decreased aqueous outflow
Features:

- Onset: third to tenth year of life
- Heredity: usually sporadic, up to 10% recessive inheritance with variable penetrance
- Signs and symptoms:
  - Pain unusual, often presents late with symptomatic visual field loss
  - Peak IOP: > 24 mm Hg without treatment
  - Cornea: Diameter: < 11 mm (no buphthalmos, no corneal edema)
  - Optic nerve head: pressure distension/cup enlargement with diffuse rim damage
  - Gonioscopy: open-angle
    - poorly differentiated structures, trabeculodysgenesis
    - anterior insertion of the iris

2.1.3 - GLAUCOMA ASSOCIATED WITH CONGENITAL ANOMALIES

a. Anidria
b. Sturge-Weber syndrome
c. Neurofibromatosis
d. Marfan syndrome
e. Pierre Robin syndrome
f. Homocystinuria
g. Goniodysgenesis: g.1 - Axenfeld-Rieger syndrome
g.2 - Peter's anomaly
h. Lowe's syndrome
i. Microspherophakia
j. Microcornea
k. Rubella
l. Chromosomal abnormalities
m. Broad thumb syndrome
n. Persistent hyperplastic primary vitreous

2.2 - PRIMARY OPEN-ANGLE GLAUCOMAS

The open-angle glaucomas are chronic, progressive optic neuropathies, that have in common characteristic morphological changes at the optic nerve head and retinal nerve fibre layer in the absence of other ocular disease or congenital anomalies. Progressive retinal ganglion cells death and visual field loss are associated with these changes.
The relative risk for POAG rises continuously with the level of the intra-ocular pressure (IOP), and there is no evidence of a threshold IOP for the onset of the condition. It is presumed that risk factors other than IOP have a relatively greater importance if there is glaucomatous optic neuropathy at the lower (statistically 'normal') pressure levels. POAG has been arbitrarily subdivided into High Pressure and Normal Pressure disease to reflect this, even though they may represent a spectrum of optic neuropathies variably sensitive to the IOP.

Risk Factors associated with increased prevalence of glaucoma damage

Glaucomatous damage in the fellow eye
Level of intra-ocular pressure, as confirmed in all recent trials (see Ch. Introduction II)
Age
Race
Thin cornea
Pseudoexfoliation
Myopia > 4 diopters
Vascular risk factors:

- Local:
  disc hemorrhage, associated also with worsening of damage
  peripapillary atrophy, associated also with worsening of damage

- Systemic:
  cerebral disease
  cardiovascular disease
  vasospasm: cold hands and feet
  Raynaud's phenomena
  migraine
  systemic hypotension with nocturnal pressure drops
  low perfusion pressure
  hypercholesterolemia / hyperlipidemia.

Family history of glaucoma in first degree relatives
Diabetes Mellitus: the role is controversial

For detailed references a recent review on Evidence - Based glaucoma knowledge is suggested, as well as references in the Introduction Chapter[1].

Supplementary investigations

I - If findings do not match, central corneal thickness (CCT) can be useful to evaluate the IOP applanation value (see Ch. 1.1). There is accumulating evidence that a correction factor needs to be incorporated into the readings taken by Goldmann applanation tonometry according to CCT.
II - MRI scan of the pituitary gland and ONH indicated if there is an atypical appearance of the optic disc or the visual field defects are suspicious of neurological disease or disc and visual field findings are inconsistent.
III - Doppler ultrasound of supra-aortic vessels, particularly when disc and visual field findings are inconsistant with the IOP.

2.2.1 - PRIMARY JUVENILE GLAUCOMA

Etiology: Unknown
Pathomechanism: Decreased aqueous outflow
Features:
- Onset: tenth to 35th year of life
- Heredity: family history may be present. Genes associated with primary juvenile glaucoma have been identified on chromosome 1 (1q21-q31) and MYOC [2,3]
- Signs and symptoms:
  - Asymptomatic
  - Peak IOP ≥ 21 mm Hg without treatment (diurnal tension curve)
  - Optic nerve head: Diffuse rim damage typical. Any type of ONH glaucomatos defect is possible
  - Nerve fiber layer: typical diffuse defects
  - Visual field: glaucomatous defects may be present
  - Gonioscopy: wide open anterior chamber angle

2.2.2 - PRIMARY JUVENILE GLAUCOMA SUSPECT

Etiology: Unknown
Pathomechanism: Unknown
Features:
- Onset: tenth to 35th year of life
- No structural or functional defects with normal optic disc, nerve fiber layer and visual field
- Heredity: family history may be present. Genes associated with primary juvenile glaucoma have been identified on chromosome 1 (1q21-q31) and MYOC mutation[2-3]
  - AND

Either I:
- Peak pressure: ≥ 31mm Hg (without treatment)

Or II:
- at least two of the following risk factors:
  - a) peak pressure 22 mm Hg to 30 mm Hg
  - b) IOP difference > 4 mm Hg between the two eyes
  - c) family history of glaucoma
  - d) manifest juvenile glaucoma in the opposite eye

2.2.3 - PRIMARY OPEN-ANGLE GLAUCOMA/High Pressure Glaucoma (POAG/HPG)

See Ch. Introduction and 2.2
Etiology: Unknown
Pathomechanism: Unknown. TIGR and MYOC mutations may be associated[2,3]
Features:
- Onset: from the 35th year of age onwards
- Signs and symptoms:
  - Asymptomatic until field loss advanced
  - IOP > 21 mm Hg without treatment (diurnal tension curve)
  - Optic nerve head: acquired characteristic glaucomatous damage and/or retinal nerve fiber layer changes (diffuse or localized defects)
  - Visual field: usually detectable glaucomatous defects corresponding to the optic disc damage may be present
  - Gonioscopy: open anterior chamber angle (not occludable, no goniodysgenesis). See Ch. 1.2 and Ch. 2.4.3.

2.2.4 - PRIMARY OPEN-ANGLE GLAUCOMA SUSPECT (POAG/HPG SUSPECT)

See also Ch. Introduction and Ch. 2.2

Etiology: Unknown

Pathomechanism: Unknown

Features:

- Visual field and/or optic disc and/or nerve fiber layer normal or suspicious, with at least one being suspicious
- Peak IOP > 21 mm Hg < 30 mm Hg without treatment (diurnal tension curve)
- Gonioscopy: open anterior chamber angle
- Risk factors to be considered:
  - IOP difference > 4 mm Hg between the two eyes
  - Peak IOP value
  - Any other vascular risk factor for glaucomatous optic neuropathy (See Ch. 2.2)
  - POAG in fellow eye
  - AION in fellow eye

Note

Pseudoexfoliation and pigment dispersion are risk factors for secondary open-angle glaucoma.

High IOP is associated with, but not proven to be a causal factor of vein occlusion, especially in patients with high blood pressure, hypercholesterolemia or obesity.

2.2.5 - PRIMARY OPEN-ANGLE GLAUCOMA/Normal-Pressure Glaucoma (POAG/NPG)

See Ch. Introduction and Ch. 2.2

Etiology: Unknown

Pathomechanism: Unknown. Optineurin mutation has been found in families with NPG

Features:

- Onset: from the 35th year onwards
- Signs and symptoms:
  - Asymptomatic until field loss advanced
  - Peak IOP < 22 mm Hg without treatment (diurnal tension curve)
  - Optic nerve head damage typical of glaucoma
  - Disc hemorrhage
  - Visual field defect typical of glaucoma; common paracentral defects
  - Gonioscopy: open anterior chamber angle (exclude intermittent angle-closure; see Ch. 2.4.3)
  - No history or signs of other eye disease or steroid use.

Consider central corneal thickness if findings do not match (see Ch. 1.1)

2.2.6 - POAG/Normal-Pressure Glaucoma Suspect (POAG/NPG-SUSPECT)

Etiology: Unknown

Pathomechanism: Unknown

Features:

- Signs and symptoms:
  - Visual field: normal or suspicious
  - Optic disc and/or nerve fibre layer: findings not diagnostic of, but compatible with, the diagnosis of glaucoma
  - Peak IOP: < 22 mm Hg without treatment (diurnal tension curve or refeated measurements)
  - Gonioscopy: open anterior chamber angle (exclude intermittent angle-closure see Ch. 2.4.3)
- Risk factors to be considered:
  - IOP difference > 4 mm Hg between the two eyes
  - Any other vascular risk factor for glaucomatous optic neuropathy (See Ch. 2.2)
  - NPG in fellow eye

Consider corneal thickness if findings do not match (see Ch. 1.1)

2.2.7 - OCULAR HYPERTENSION (OH)

Etiology: Unknown
Pathomechanism: Unknown
Features:

Signs and symptoms:

- Peak IOP > 21 mm Hg without treatment (diurnal curve)
- Visual field: normal
- Optic disc and retinal nerve fibre layer: normal
- Gonioscopy: open anterior chamber angle (exclude intermittent angle-closure. See Ch. 2.4.3)
- No history or signs of other eye disease or steroid use.
- Other risk factors: none

High IOP is associated with, but not proven to be causal of vein occlusion, especially in patients with high blood pressure, hypercholesterolemia or obesity.

Consider corneal thickness if findings do not match. See Ch. 1.1

Although in the past it has been used as a diagnosis and still is usually separated for research and classification purposes, the term ocular hypertension (OH) should be used just to indicate that the IOP is consistenly outside two standard deviations from the normal mean, with all other ocular findings within normal limits.

Elevated IOP causing progressive typical glaucomatous optic neuropathy and visual field loss, caused by ophthalmological or extraocular disease(s), drugs and treatments. Assessment of the glaucomatous damage to visual function, including visual field staging, may be difficult because of the underlying ophthalmological diseases or complex clinical picture.

The following classification is primarily based on pathophysiologic mechanisms. Distinct clinical glaucoma types are discussed at the corresponding point of the mechanistic classification.

When no etiology and pathomechanism are evident, a primary glaucoma should be considered.

In secondary Open-angle Glaucomas the anterior chamber-angle is open for over 270°.

In several forms of secondary glaucoma pathomechanisms leading to both secondary open-angle and angle-closure glaucoma are combined. Since the number of the combinations is very high, in each case individual evaluation is necessary.

2.3.1 - SECONDARY OPEN-ANGLE GLAUCOMAS CAUSED BY OPHTHALMOLOGICAL CONDITIONS

2.3.1.1 - Pseudoexfoliation Glaucoma (PEX)[4,5]

Etiology: Pseudoexfoliative material, an abnormal fibrillo-granular protein, and pigment accumulate in the trabecular meshwork, where TM function decreases. Similar material has been identified in the conjuntiva and body parts outside the eye. Why many eyes with pseudoexfoliation do not have glaucoma is not known.
Pathomechanism: Reduction of the trabecular outflow owing to the pseudoexfoliative material.
Features:

- Onset: usually older than 60 years
- Frequency: large racial variations
- Asymptomatic until visual field loss advanced
- One or both eyes affected, often bilateral and asymmetrical
- Sign and symptoms:
  - IOP: >21 mm Hg, frequently higher than in average POAG cases
  - Visual field loss as in POAG; frequently severe at least in one eye
  - Slit lamp examination: dandruff-like exfoliation material on the pupil border and on the surface of the anterior lens capsule except the central zone, better visualized after pupillary dilation. The pupillary collarette is irregular and typically has a moth-eaten appearance.

Frequently associated with nuclear cataract, pigmentary loss from the central or mid-iris, pigment granules in the angle. When pigment accumulates along an ondulating line on or anterior to Schwalbe's line, it is called Sampaolesi's line. Loose zonules are frequent with occasional phacodonesis and lens subluxation.
Narrow or closed-angle is relatively common.

2.3.1.2 - Pigmentary Glaucoma[5,6]

Etiology: Melanin granules accumulate in the trabecular meshwork, where TM function decreases.
Pathomechanism: Reduction of the trabecular outflow owing to melanin granules. According to the theory of 'reverse pupillary block' the iris works as a valve resulting in IOP higher in the anterior chamber than in the posterior chamber, causing peripheral posterior bowing of the iris. Melanin granules are released from the iris as a result of rubbing between the zonules and the posterior surface of the iris.

Features:

Onset: typically third to fifth decades

Frequency: 1-1.5 % of the total glaucoma cases, mostly Caucasians, more in myopic males

One or both eyes

Sign and symptoms:

Uncommonly mild to moderate pain during acute episodes of IOP rise. Haloes around lights.

IOP: > 21 mm Hg, characteristically with large variations. Significant increase may occur after exercise, pupillary dilation or blinking. Gradual decrease of IOP with age over 60 years has been reported.

Slit lamp examination: deep anterior chamber, midperipheral iris pigment epithelial atrophy with radial pattern especially well visible with retroillumination. Pigment dispersed on the trabecular meshwork, Schwalbe's line, the iris surface, the lens equator and on the corneal endothelium, where often shapes itself as a central, vertical spindle (Krukenberg's spindle). Dim light in the examination room is recommended, in order to enhance the observation of the peripheral iris shape. UBM examination is often helpful to diagnose reverse pupillary block.

2.3.1.3 - Lens-induced Secondary Open-Angle Glaucoma

Etiology: Obstruction of the trabecular meshwork by lens proteins and/or inflammatory cells induced by lens proteins.

Pathomechanism:

- Lens proteins from a mature or hypermature cataract with intact capsule (phacolytic glaucoma)
- Lens particles from a traumatically or surgically injured lens (lens particle glaucoma)
- Granulomatous inflammation of the TM after uneventful ECCE when the fellow eye was already operated and its lens proteins sensitized the immune system (phacoanaphylactic glaucoma)

Features:

Age of onset and acute or chronic course depend on the pathomechanism

Sign and symptoms:

Often painful with redness and inflammation

IOP > 21 mm Hg

Slit lamp examination: injured lens and/or cataract or after ECCE, with or without iritis

2.3.1.4 - Glaucoma associated with intraocular haemorrhage

Etiology: Obstruction of the trabecular meshwork by rigid red blood cells (ghost cell glaucoma, Sickle cell disease) or by a large quantity of normal red blood cells (hyphaema).

Pathomechanism: Red blood cells (ghost cells) from an old vitreous hemorrhage, via a ruptured anterior hyaloid face, or from the iris (for example trauma, intraocular surgery) obstruct the trabecular meshwork

Features:

Sign and symptoms:

Pain, redness, recurrences possible

IOP > 21 mm Hg

2.3.1.5 - Uveitic Glaucoma

Etiology: Several forms of anterior and intermediate uveitis can cause unilateral or bilateral obstruction of the trabecular meshwork. The most frequent conditions are juvenile rheumatoid arthritis, Fuchs' heterochromic iridocyclitis, Posner-Schlossman syndrome (glaucomatocyclitic crisis), herpes simplex, herpes zoster, syphilis, sarcoidosis, Behçet disease, sympathetic ophthalmia, pars planitis.

Pathomechanism: Obstruction and edema of the trabecular meshwork caused by inflammatory cells, precipitates, debris, secondary scarring and neovascularization of the chamber angle. Secondary angle-closure glaucoma due to synechiae can also develop.

Features:

Onset depends on underlying condition. Any age

Sign and symptoms:

Pain, redness, photophobia, decreased vision are possible.

IOP > 21 mm Hg. Some forms are associated with wide oscillations or periodic rise of IOP.

2.3.1.6 - Glaucoma due to intraocular tumors

Etiology: Reduced aqueous humour outflow due to primary or secondary intraocular (anterior segment) tumors
Pathomechanism: Compression or tumor extension to the trabecular meshwork and/or outflow channels. Trabecular meshwork obstruction due to tumor related inflammation, tumor necrosis, hemorrhage and pigment dispersion. (Secondary angle-closure glaucoma may also develop)
Features:
- Sign and symptoms:
  - IOP > 21 mm Hg
  - Onset and clinical picture highly variable, combining evidence for both the tumor and the glaucoma

2.3.1.7 - Glaucoma associated with retinal detachment

Etiology: Although retinal detachment is usually associated with lower than normal IOP, the same disease processes can also cause both reduced trabecular outflow and retinal detachment
Pathomechanism: Neovascularization, proliferative retinopathy, scarring, pigment dispersion and inflammation (e.g. photoreceptor sensitization). Cases in which surgery for retinal detachment causes glaucoma are discussed in part 2.5. See also Ch. 2.3.1.8
Features:
- Sign and symptoms:
  - IOP > 21 mm Hg
  - Redness, pain are possible
  - Retinal detachment is present

Note
In general, retinal detachment is associated with lower than normal IOP.
Surgery for retinal detachment repair can cause glaucoma. See also Ch. 2.3.2.2.

2.3.1.8 - Open-Angle Glaucoma due to ocular trauma

Ocular trauma leads to glaucoma by several different mechanisms. The secondary traumatic glaucomas can be caused by both open-angle and angle-closure pathomechanisms. To identify the etiology one must carefully evaluate all traumatic damage to the eye.
Etiology: Reduced trabecular outflow due to traumatic changes of the trabecular meshwork
Pathomechanism: Scarring and inflammation of the trabecular meshwork, obstruction by red blood cells and debris, lens induced glaucoma, angle recession. Positive steroid responsiveness to be also considered (see Ch. 2.3.2.1).
Features:
- Highly variable
- Signs and symptoms:
  - Redness, pain, decreased vision, or no symptoms
  - IOP > 21 mm Hg. Elevated intraocular pressure can be present immediately, but slow elevation occuring months, or up to decades later are also possible.
  - Slit lamp examination: chemical burns, hyphema, traumatic cataract, swollen lens, uveitis, angle recession, ruptured iris sphincter.

2.3.2 - IATROGENIC SECONDARY OPEN-ANGLE GLAUCOMAs

2.3.2.1 - Glaucoma due to corticosteroid treatment

Etiology: Reduced trabecular outflow due to trabecular changes caused by corticosteroids (TIGR/MYOC protein)[2-3]
Pathomechanism: Topical as well as high dose and long-term systemic corticosteroid therapy induces changes in the trabecular extracellular material (glycoproteins) which leads to decreased outflow facility. Usually pressure elevation is reversible if the corticosteroid is stopped. A modification of the TIGR gene was demonstrated.
Features:
- Individual, hereditary susceptibility can occur. Myopic, diabetic subjects and POAG Patients may be more susceptible

Signs and symptoms:

No pain, no redness, corneal edema is possible

IOP > 21 mm Hg

Typical glaucomatous optic nerve head and visual field damage if the disease is long-standing

2.3.2.2 - Secondary Open-Angle Glaucoma due to ocular surgery and laser

Ocular surgery can cause secondary open-angle glaucoma by some of the mechanisms discussed above: pigmentary loss from uveal tissue, lens material, haemorrhage, uveitis and trauma. See also ch.s 2.3.1.1 to 2.3.2.1

Etiology: Reduced trabecular outflow

Pathomechanism:

- Viscoelastic materials, inflammatory debris, intra-operative application of alpha-chymotrypsin, lens particles, vitreous in the anterior chamber after cataract surgery, prostaglandin release. IOP elevation is usually transient.
- Acute onset secondary IOP elevation after Nd:YAG laser iridotomy, capsulotomy and argon laser trabeculoplasty. Usually transient, within the first 24 hours, most frequent in the first 4 hours after treatment.
- Emulsion of silicone oil implanted intravitreally enters the anterior chamber and is partially phagocytosed by macrophages and accumulates in the trabecular meshwork (especially in the upper quadrant).
- Uveitis -glaucoma- hyphema (UGH) syndrome. Episodic onset, associated with anterior chamber pseudophakia.

IOP elevation is induced by recurrent iris root bleeding and anterior uveitis.

Features:

Sign and symptoms:

Pain, redness, corneal edema are possible

IOP > 21 mm Hg

Visual field loss when IOP elevation is sufficient/prolonged

2.3.3 - SECONDARY OPEN-ANGLE GLAUCOMA CAUSED BY EXTRAOCULAR CONDITIONS

2.3.3.1 - Glaucoma caused by increased episcleral venous pressure

Etiology: Increase of the episcleral venous pressure which causes reduced trabecular outflow and elevated intraocular pressure

Pathomechanism: Episcleral, orbital or general causes for reduced episcleral venous outflow:

* Dural shunts
* Chemical burn, radiation damage of the episcleral veins
* Endocrine orbitopathy
* Orbital (retrobulbar) tumour, pseudotumour,
* Orbital phlebitis
* Orbital or intracranial arteriovenous fistula
* Sturge-Weber syndrome
* Nevus of Ota
* Cavernous sinus thrombosis
* Jugular vein obstruction (radical neck dissections)
* Superior vena cava obstruction
* Pulmonary venous obstruction
* Idiopathic forms

Features:

Onset can be acute

Signs and symptoms:

Wide variations of clinical features

IOP > 21 mm Hg

Dilated, congested episcleral veins, chemosis, facial lymphoedema, orbital bruit

Vascular bruits in case of A/V fistulae

Primary angle-closure is appositional or synechial closure of the anterior chamber angle due to a number of possible mechanisms. This may result in raised IOP and may cause structural changes in the eye.
The principal argument to strictly separate primary angle-closure glaucoma from primary open-angle glaucoma is the initial therapeutic approach (i.e. iridotomy or iridectomy) and the possible late complications (synechial closure of chamber angle) or the complications resulting when this type of glaucoma undergoes filtering surgery (uveal effusion, malignant glaucoma)[7,8].

Angle-closure glaucomas are clinically divided into the acute and chronic forms. The pathogenesis is however multifold and varies according to the underlying condition. By definition, in acute angle-closure, the chamber angle is closed by iridocorneal apposition that can be reversed, whereas in chronic angle-closure, the angle-closure is irreversible due to peripheral anterior synechiae.

PROVOCATIVE TESTS

In general provocative tests for angle-closure provide little additional information since even when negative they may not rule out the potential for angle-closure. In addition they may be hazardous, triggering an acute angle-closure attack even while the patient is monitored.

2.4.1 - PRIMARY ANGLE-CLOSURE (PAC)

Angle-closure is defined on the basis of findings at gonioscopy

Mechanisms of primary angle-closure[9,10]
It is always important to exclude secondary causes of narrow or closed-angles such as a phakomorphic or inflammatory mechanism. In isometropic eyes this can be helped by comparing axial anterior chamber depths. A-scan or UBM may be helpful in defining the anatomical relationships and measure axial length, AC depth and lens thickness or PC configuration. In primary angle-closure these will be the same in each eye.

a) Pupillary block mechanism

A component of pupillary block accounts for most cases of acute, intermittent and chronic primary angle-closure.
In pupillary block, the flow of aqueous from the posterior chamber through the pupil to the anterior chamber is impeded causing the pressure in the posterior chamber to become higher than the pressure in the anterior chamber. As a result, the peripheral iris, which is thinner than the central iris, bows forward and comes into contact with the trabecular meshwork and Schwalbe's line.
This circular obstruction of the trabecular outflow leads to a rise of IOP up to levels of 50-80 mm Hg; when this occurs within a few hours, it causes the symptoms and signs of acute angle-closure(AAC).
The increased resistance to transpupillary aqueous flow is caused by apposition of the posterior surface of the iris to the anterior surface of the lens.
The pupillary block mechanism may be precipitated during mid-dilation of the pupil or in conditions where the constrictor and dilator muscles of the pupil are acting together, physiologically as in reading in poor light or pharmacologically, such as with miotic therapy and concomitant dilator muscle stimulation by phenylephrine (the Mapstone provocation test)[5]. In most cases, the predisposition to pupil block is created by a narrow anterior segment and the age-related increase of lens volume (see Ch. 2.5.1 and 2.5.3).
The prevalence of PAC is higher in hyperopia, in elderly patients, in diabetics, women and in some races (especially Sino-Mongolians)[8,9].

b) Plateau-iris mechanism

The isolated plateau iris mechanism causes angle-closure by direct obliteration of the chamber angle recess, crowded by the iris base when the pupil is dilated. This can occur only with one or more of the following:
(1) the tissue of the peripheral iris is thick (iris rolls)
(2) the iris base inserts anteriorly, leaving only a very narrow ciliary band, or inserts at the scleral spur
(3) the ciliary processes are displaced anteriorly in the posterior chamber and push the iris base into the chamber angle.
(4) the iris profile is almost flat from the perifery to the far periphery, where it becomes very steep, creating an extremely narrow angle recess.

The iris root position and the posterior chamber anatomy can be confirmed by ultrasound biomicroscopy.
It is clear from these descriptions why the isolated plateau iris mechanism is not altered by iridectomy.

The pure plateau iris syndrome, causing angle-closure despite a patent iridotomy, is extremely rare compared with pupillary block. Both mechanisms, however, may coincide when "plateau iris configuration" is present. This latter condition is relatively common. The pure form of plateau iris syndrome can only be proven by the occurrence of acute angle-closure triggered by mydriasis despite a patent iridectomy and a centrally deep anterior chamber.

Due to the above mechanisms, in all combined pupillary block/plateau iris cases iridotomy or iridectomy should be performed first. Plateau iris can be treated by argon laser iridoplasty and/or miotic therapy, preferably with topical sympatholytics like dapiprazole or thymoxamine. Strong miotics are to be avoided, because they cause anterior rotation of the ciliary body. Ideally, treatment should be instituted before synechial closure of the angle occurs (see Ch. 4.4.1).

c) Lens mechanism

Large and/or anteriorly placed cristalline lens can predispose per se to angle-closure and be a factor in worsening pupillary block. It can also cause secondary angle-closure glaucoma (see Ch. 2.5.1 and 2.5.3.).

d) Creeping angle-closure mechanism

Some cases of chronic angle-closure glaucoma result from synechial closure of the chamber angle, caused by a previous acute angle-closure 'attack', while creeping angle-closure is probably a primary event. The iris base 'creeps' on to the trabecular meshwork forming irreversible peripheral anterior synechiae (PAS). The IOP usually rises when more than half of the angle is obstructed. It is not yet clear whether creeping angle-closure is the consequence of undiagnosed intermittent angle-closure or a consequence of chronic miotic therapy causing worsening relative pupillary block. This form seems to be more frequent in Asians.

e) Posterior aqueous misdirection mechanism

In rare cases posterior aqueous misdirection can be the cause of primary angle-closure, mostly resulting in chronic IOP elevation. In these cases, usually younger or middle aged women, the ciliary processes come into contact with the lens equator, and/or a firm zonule/posterior capsule diaphragm, causing misdirection of aqueous into the vitreous[8,9]. As a consequence, the lens/iris diaphragm is pushed forward and occludes the chamber angle. Eyes predisposed to posterior aqueous misdirection often have narrow anterior chambers (peripheral and axial) and hypermetropia. After iridotomy or iridectomy, the use of miotics raises the IOP, whereas the use of cycloplegics reduces the IOP. This 'inverse' or 'paradoxical' reaction to parasympathomimetics should be tested only after iridotomy has been performed. Ultrasound biomicroscopy can demonstrate abnormal posterior chamber anatomy in these rare cases (see Ch. 2.5.3).

<u>Systemic drugs and angle-closure:</u>
Systemic drugs which may induce angle-closure in pre-disposed individuals are phenothiazines and their derivatives, tricyclic and non-tricyclic antidepressants, monoamine oxidase inhibitors, antihistamines, anti-Parkinson drugs, some minor tranquilizers, parasympatholytic and sympathomimetic agent (see Ch. 1.4).

Systemic Risk factors for primary angle-closure[8,11]

- Female
- Family history if primary angle-closure
- Necessity of using sympathomimetics or sympatholytics
- Race: Eskimo, Asians

Primary angle-closure. Descriptions of Glaucoma types[12,13]

Primary angle-closure glaucoma is divided into 3 subtypes:

- Acute Angle-Closure Glaucoma (AACG)
- Intermittent Angle-Closure Glaucoma (IACG)
- Chronic Angle-Closure Glaucoma (CACG)

Etiology: iridotrabecular contact and/or adhesion
Pathomechanism: decreased aqueous outflow due to TM occlusion
Features: angle-closed at gonioscopy, without a discernible cause

2.4.1.1 - Acute Angle-Closure Glaucoma (AACG)

Etiology: circumferential iris apposition to the trabecular meshwork with rapid and excessive increase in intraocular pressure (IOP) that does not resolve spontaneously.
Pathomechanism: see Ch. 2.4.1
Features:

Signs:

IOP elevated often to 50-80 mm Hg
Decreased visual acuity
Corneal edema, initially mostly epithelial edema
Shallow or flat peripheral anterior chamber
Peripheral iris pushed forward and in contact with Schwalbe's line.
Gonioscopy: angle-closure 360 degrees
Pupil mid-dilated and reduced or no reactivity
Venous congestion and ciliary injection
Fundus: disc edema, with venous congestion and splinter hemorrhages, or the disc may be normal or show glaucomatous escavation
Bradycardia or arrhythmia
Gonioscopy clues from the other eye

Symptoms:

Blurred vision
"Halos" around lights
Pain
Frontal headache of variable degree on the side of the affected eye
Nausea and vomiting, occasionally
Palpitations, abdominal cramps, occasionally

2.4.1.2 - Intermittent Angle-Closure Glaucoma (IACG)

Etiology: similar but milder clinical manifestations than AACG, it resolves spontaneously.
Pathomechanism: see ch. 2.4.1
Features:

Signs:

May vary according to amount of appositional closure of chamber angle and mimic acute angle-closure in a mild form. When not on miotics, pupil is round and reactive

The optic disc rim may show atrophy with an afferent pupillary defect

Symptoms:

Mild, intermittent symptoms of acute angle-closure type

2.4.1.3 - Chronic Angle-Closure Glaucoma (CACG)

Etiology: permanent synechial closure of any extent of the chamber angle as confirmed by indentation gonioscopy.
Pathomechanism: see Ch. 2.4.1
Features:

Signs:

Peripheral anterior synechiae of any degree at gonioscopy
IOP elevated to a variable degree depending on the extent of angle-closure, above 21 mm Hg
Visual acuity according to functional status (may be normal)
Damage of optic nerve head compatible with glaucoma

Visual field defects "typical" of chronic glaucoma may be present

Superimposed intermittent or acute angle-closure possible

Symptoms:

Visual disturbances according to functional states
Usually no pain; sometimes discomfort
Transient "haloes" when intermittent closure of the total circumference causes acute IOP elevations

2.4.2 - STATUS POST ACUTE ANGLE-CLOSURE ATTACK

Etiology: previous episode of acute angle-closure attack
Pathomechanism: see Ch. 2.4.1
Features:

Signs:

Patchy iris atrophy
Iris torsion/spiralling
Posterior synechiae
Pupil either poorly reactive or non reactive
"Glaukomflecken" of the anterior lens surface
Peripheral anterior synechiae on gonioscopy
Endothelial cell count can be decreased

2.4.3 - THE "OCCLUDABLE" ANGLE; ACR (Angle-Closure Risk)

Etiology: pupillary block, plateau iris or lens; each component plays different roles in different eyes
Pathomechanism: see Ch. 2.4.1
Features:

Signs:

Iridotrabecular apposition and/or PAS
IOP elevation may be present

Fellow eye of acute angle-closure attack
Fellow eye of documented non-secondary angle-closure

OCCLUDABLE ANGLE:

"Occludable" is not an objective evidence - based finding but a clinical diagnosis. Since an occludable angle is defined as one that has high risk of closure, it must be treated with iridotomy/iridectomy to eliminate the pupillary block component.

If the iridotomy is patent, should the angle not deepen, iridoplasty may be considered, depending on the main mechanism underlying the risk of angle occlusion. Topical pilocarpine or dapripazole treatment should be considered whilst awaiting iridotomy / iridectomy.

NARROW ANGLE:

The term "narrow angle glaucoma" does not describe whether the main cause of IOP increase is primary impairment of trabecular outflow facility or mechanical obstruction of the trabeculum by iris apposition or synechial closure. Both mechanisms may co-exist in an eye with a narrow anterior chamber angle. Therefore the term "narrow angle glaucoma" should be avoided as non-specific.

If an occludable angle is present (i.e. in addition to POAG), this should be referred as POAG with an occludable angle or with risk of angle-closure (See also Ch. 2.4.3).

If intermittent angle-closure is present, the condition should be considered, and treated, as angle-closure glaucoma. If a case of POAG has a narrow angle, it should be labeled as POAG with narrow angle approach.

2.5 - SECONDARY ANGLE-CLOSURE GLAUCOMAS

Angle-closure glaucomas are clinically divided into the acute and chronic forms. The pathogenesis is however many fold and varies according to the underlying condition. By definition, in acute angle-closure, the chamber angle is closed by iridocorneal apposition that can be reversed, whereas in chronic secondary angle-closure, the angle-closure is irreversible due to peripheral anterior synechiae.

2.5.1 - SECONDARY ANGLE-CLOSURE GLAUCOMAS WITH PUPILLARY BLOCK

Etiology: The following is a limited list of other etiology for relative or absolute pupillary block:

- Swollen lens (cataract, traumatic cataract)
- Anterior lens dislocation (trauma, zonular laxity; Weil-Marchesani's syndrome, Marfans's syndrome etc.)
- Posterior synechiae, seclusion or occlusion of the pupil
- Protruding vitreous face or intravitreal silicone oil in aphakia
- Microspherophakia
- Miotic-induced pupillary block (also the lens moves forward)
- IOL-induced pupillary block (ACL, anteriorly dislocated PCL)[14]

Pathomechanism: Pupillary block pushes the iris forward to occlude the angle. In iritis or iridocyclitis, the development of posterior synechiae may lead to absolute pupillary block with consequent forward bowing of the iris or "iris bombé". Acute secondary angle-closure glaucoma may result.

Features:

- IOP > 21 mmHg
- Disc features compatible with glaucoma

2.5.2 - SECONDARY ANGLE-CLOSURE GLAUCOMA WITH ANTERIOR "PULLING" MECHANISM WITHOUT PUPILLARY BLOCK

Etiology:

- Neovascular glaucoma where the iridotrabecular fibrovascular membrane is induced by ocular microvascular disease
- Iridocorneal Endothelial (I.C.E.) Syndrome, with progressive endothelial membrane formation and progressive iridotrabecular adhesion
- Peripheral anterior synechiae, due to prolonged primary angle-closure glaucoma; this is theoretically a primary glaucoma.
- Epithelial and fibrous ingrowth after anterior segment surgery or penetrating trauma
- Inflammatory membrane
- After argon laser trabeculoplasty (ALT), early and late peripheral anterior synechiae and endothelial membrane covering the trabecular meshwork
- Aniridia
- Endothelial Posterior polymorphous dystrophy

Pathomechanism: The trabecular meshwork is obstructed by iris tissue or a membrane. The iris and/or a membrane is progressively pulled forward to occlude the angle.

Features:

- IOP > 21 mmHg
- Disc features compatible with glaucoma

2.5.3 - SECONDARY ANGLE-CLOSURE GLAUCOMA WITH POSTERIOR 'PUSHING' MECHANISM WITHOUT PUPILLARY BLOCK

2.5.3.1 - Aqueous misdirection (ciliary block or malignant) glaucoma

Etiology: Angle-closure is caused by the ciliary body and iris rotating forward
Pathomechanism:
* The lens may be proportionally abnormally large or swollen, as in phacomorphic mechanism
* Aqueous humour accumulates in the vitreous body (posterior aqueous humour misdirection) or behind and around the crystalline lens (perilenticular misdirection) or behind the iridocapsular diaphragm or posterior chamber intraocular lens (PCL) after extracapsular cataract surgery, with or without PCL implantation (retrocapsular misdirection)[12]
* Frequently precipitated by ocular surgery and flat anterior chamber[8]
* Predisposition may be similar in both eyes particularly in small eyes

2.5.3.2 - Iris and ciliary body cysts , intraocular tumors

2.5.3.3 - Silicon oil or gas implanted in the vitreous cavity[15]

2.5.3.4 - Uveal effusion[16,17] due to:

a - Inflammation as in scleritis, uveitis, HIV infection
b - Increased choroidal venous pressure as in nanophthalmos, scleral buckling, panretinal photocoagulation, central retinal vein occlusion, arterio-venous communication
c - Tumor

2.5.3.5 - Retinopathy of prematurity (stage V)

Features:

Signs and Symptoms:
- Variable discomfort, pain, redness, corneal edema
- IOP $\geq$ 21 mm Hg
- Axially shallow anterior chamber

2.5.3.6 - Congenital anomalies that can be associated with secondary glaucoma

Etiology: Familial iris hypoplasia, anomalous superficial iris vessels, aniridia, Sturge - Weber syndrome, neurofibromatosis, Marfan's syndrome, Pierre Robin syndrome, homocystinuria, goniodysgenesis, Lowe's syndrome, microcornea, microspherophakia, rubella, broad thumb syndrome, persistent hyperplastic primary vitreous
Pathomechanism: Angle-closure is caused by pushing forward the ciliary body and iris. Increase of volume of the posterior segment of the eye
Features:

Signs and Symptoms:
- IOP > 21 mm Hg
- Pain, redness, corneal edema
- Axially shallow anterior chamber
- Laser iridotomy and surgical iridectomy are not effective

Some differential diagnoses:
Acute IOP elevation with corneal edema but open-angle may result from Posner Schlossman syndrome (iridocyclitic crisis), or from endothelitis/trabeculitis (as in disciform herpetic keratitis).
Neovascular glaucoma may be associated with an open or closed-angle and may mimic some signs and the symptoms of acute angle-closure.

References

1) Tuulonen A, Aiararsinen PJ, Brola E, Forsman E, Friberg K, Kaila M, Klement A, Makela M, Oskala P, Puska P, Sloranta L, Teir H, Uusitalo H, Vainio-Jylha E, Vuori ML. The finnish evidence-based guideline for open-angle glaucoma. Acta Ophthalmol Scand. 2003;81:3-18.
2) Stone EM, Fingert JH, Alward WLM et al. Identification of a gene that causes primary open-angle glaucoma. Science 1997;275(5300):668-670.
3) Lutjen-Drecoll E, May CA, Polansky JR, Johnson DH, Bloemendal H, Nguyen TD. Localized of the stress proteins aB-Crystallin and trabecular meshwork inducible glucocorticoid response protein in normal and glaucomatous trabecula meshwork. Invest Ophthalmol Vis Sci 1998;39:517-525.
4) Ritch R. Exfoliation syndrome. Curr Opic Ophthalmol 2001;12:124-130.
5) Mudumbai R, Liebmann JM, Ritch R. Combined exfoliation and pigment dispersion: an overlap syndrome. Trans Am Ophthalmol Soc 1999;97:297-314.
6) Ritch R. Pigment Dispersion Syndrome. Am J Ophthalmol 1998;126:442-445.
7) Liebmann JM, Ritch R. Complications of glaucoma surgery. In: Ritch R, Shields MB, Krupin T. The Glaucomas. St Louis, Mosby 1996;84:1703-1736.
8) Simmons RJ, Maestre FA. Malignant Glaucoma. In: Ritch R, Shields MB, Krupin T. The Glaucomas. St Louis, Mosby, 1996;39:841-855.
9) Lowe RF, Ritch R. Angle-closure glaucoma. Mechanisms and epidemiology. In: Ritch R, Shields MB, Krupin T. The Glaucomas. St Louis, Mosby, 1996;37:801-820.
10) Traverso CE. Angle-closure glaucoma. In: Duker JS and Yanoff M (eds). Ophthalmology. St. Louis, Mosby 2002: ch. 12.13.
11) Lowe RF. Primary angle-closure glaucoma: family hystories and anterior chamber depth. Br J Ophthalmol 1964;48:191-197.
12) Thygesen J, Kessing SV, Krogh E, Zibrandtsen P. The Danish Glaucoma guidelines 1997.
13) Mapstone R. Provocative tests in closed-angle glaucoma. Br J Ophthalmol 1976;60:115-117.
14) Traverso CE, Tomey KF, Gandolfo E. The glaucoma in pseudophakia. Curr Opin Ophthalmol 1996;7(2):65-71.
15) Gedde SJ Management of glaucoma after retinal detachment surgery. Curr Opin Ophthalmol 2002;13:103-109.
16) Nash RW, Lindquist T A. Bilateral angle-closure glaucoma associated with uveal effusion: Presenting sign of HIV infection. Surv Ophthalmol 1992;36:255-258.
17) Moorthy R S, Mermoud A, Baerveldt G, Minckler D S, Lee P P, Rao N A. Glaucoma associated with uveitis. Surv Ophthalmol 1997;41:361-394.

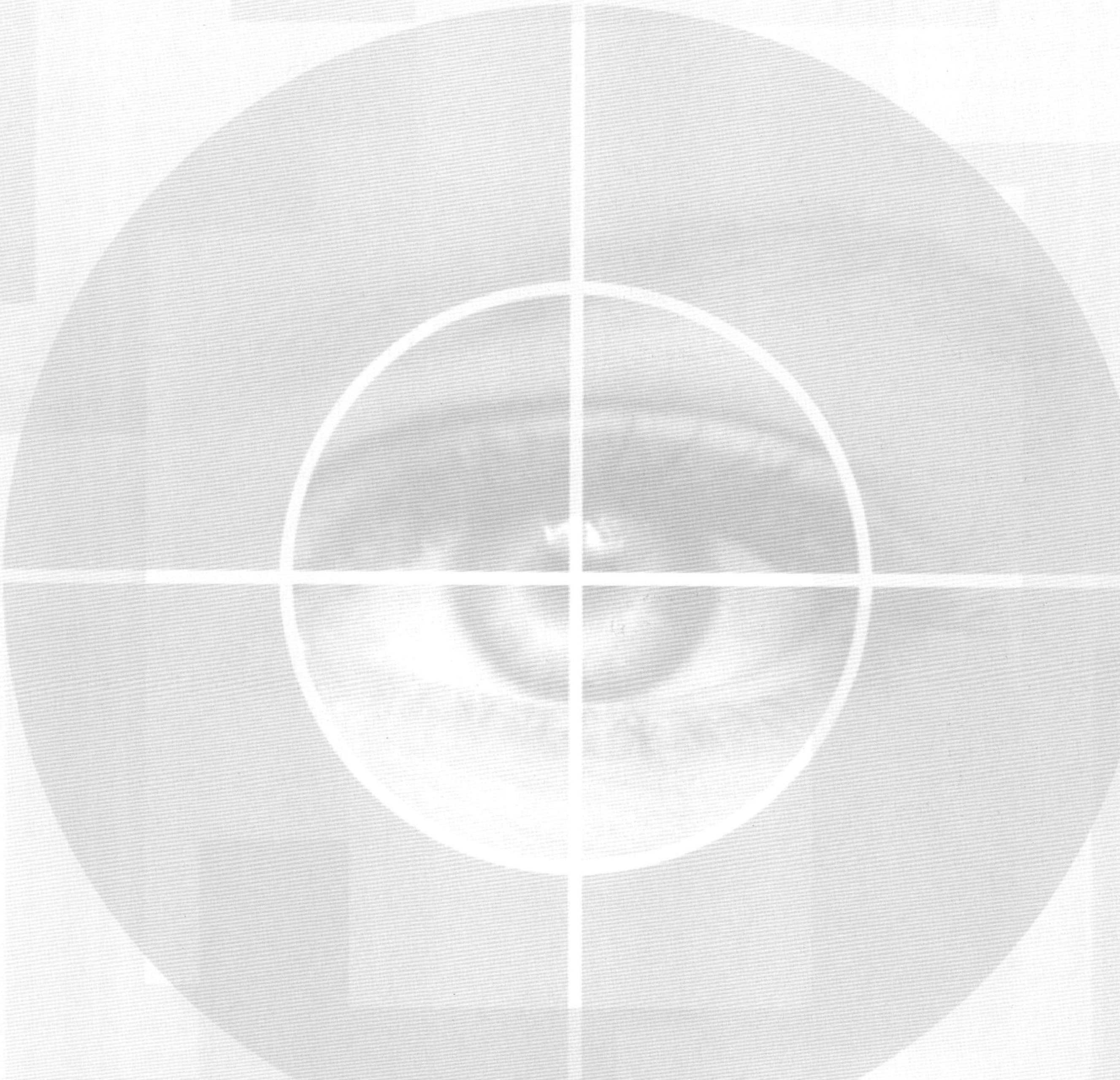

CHAPTER 3

TREATMENT PRINCIPLES and OPTIONS

• The purpose of this chapter is to give a summary overview and it is not meant to be all-inclusive
• When more than one active compound or drug category is referred to under any heading, these are listed in alphabetical order

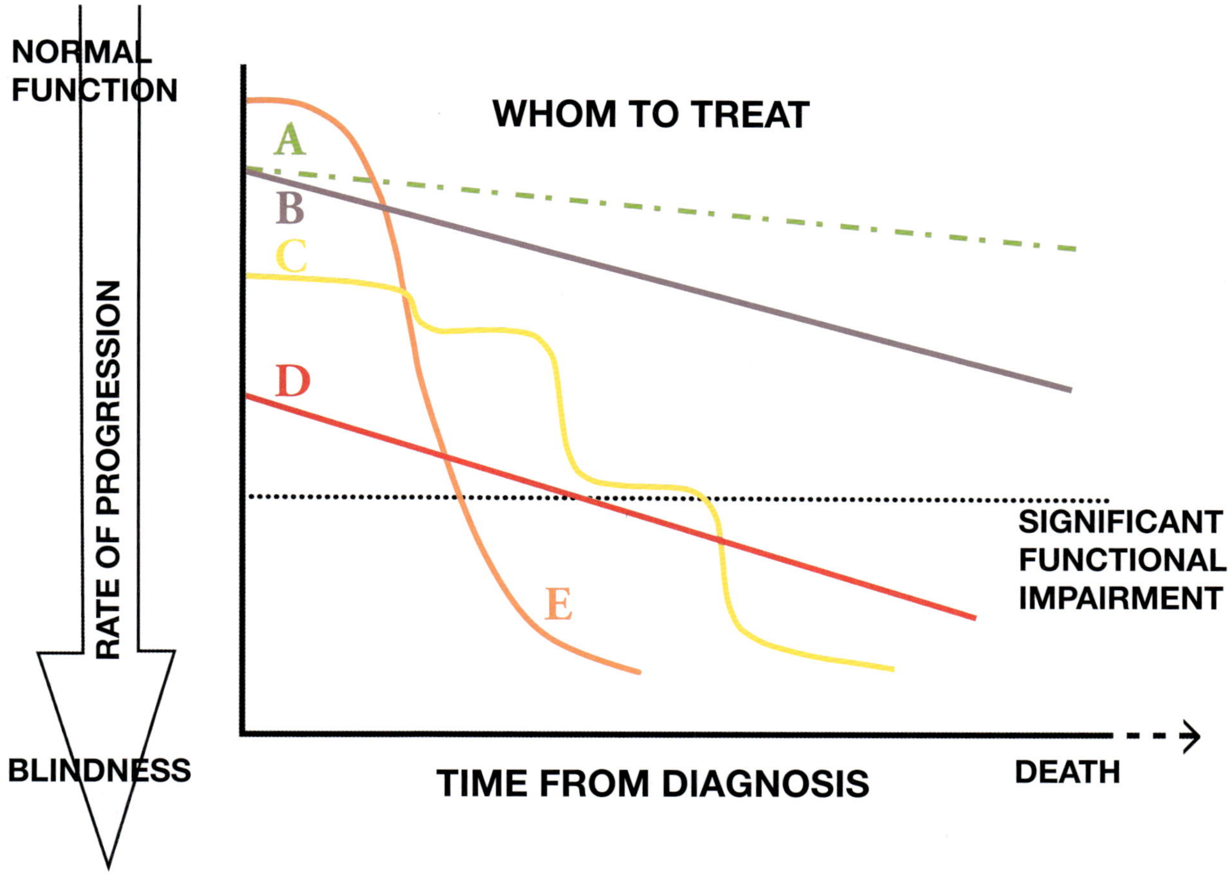

Fig. 3.1 - THE "WHOM TO TREAT" GRAPH
The rate of ganglion cell loss and consequent functional decay is different in different individuals and can vary within the same eye due to changes in time of the risk factors. To preserve the quality of life, patients must remain above the threshold of significant functional impairment. Line A represents the effect of aging alone. The patient identified by line B is worsening due to disease, but does not need treatment while those following lines C, D and E will be disabled within their lifetime unless successfully treated. To assess the likely Rate of Progression (RoP) is an important part of patient management.

The goal of glaucoma treatment is to maintain the patient's quality of life at a sustainable cost. The cost of treatment in terms of inconvenience and side effects as well as financial implications for the individual and society requires careful evaluation. The quality of life is closely linked with visual function. The treatment side effects, the dosing schedule and the constant worry about losing eye sight are all detrimental to the quality of life (see also Ch. Introduction).
Among the potential treatment options in glaucoma, *reduction of IOP, improvement of ocular blood flow, and direct neuroprotection* have been identified. Presently, the only approach proven to be efficient in preserving visual function is to lower the IOP[1-2] (see Ch. Introduction II). Current evidence indicates that alteration in blood flow may be relevant in open-angle glaucoma patients, independent of intraocular pressure[3-13]. However, because of the lack of an adequate methodology, no study that is capable of assessing the value of ocular blood flow treatment in glaucoma, has yet been designed (see also Ch. 1.6). Nevertheless, ocular blood flow is an important parameter to be considered when evaluating the direct and indirect effects of any treatment for glaucoma[5-13], as is the concept of neuroprotection.

Furthermore, blindness may occur despite treatment and individuals at appreciable risk of visual disability thus needing rigorous management must to be identified. Consequently, physicians should be advised to consider more aggressive treatment of IOP in patients suspected to have altered ocular blood flow[13]. In some patients, arterial hypotension, either drug-induced or spontaneous, is a factor to be addressed with the internist.
Neuroprotection refers to the concept of protecting ganglion cells from early death due to endo- or exotoxins or ischemia. Several experimental studies show the potential for this type of treatment in animal models on injury or in vitro. This research does not yet apply to humans. Large clinical trials are under way and results will be avaiable within 2-3 years.

A large proportion of patients with progressive glaucoma still remain undiagnosed until too late. To discover and treat those at risk of losing functionally significant vision is a more preferable task than widespread treatment of IOP per se.

It is important when selecting the medical treatment of glaucoma to understand not only the aims of therapy, but also the mode of action, side effects and contraindications of each individual medication.

There are many antiglaucoma drugs available. The choice of therapy must take into account quality of life, cost and compliance. Generally speaking, if more than two topical medications are required to control the IOP, then other forms of therapy, such as laser trabeculoplasty or surgery, should be considered.
In many patients beta-blockers have been used as the first choice of therapy since they are effective and usually well tolerated. Caution must be exercised if the patient suffers from a systemic condition such as bronchopulmonary disease or cardiac arhythmia, since the systemic absorption of these drugs may cause relevant adverse systemic effects. If the first choice medication alone does not control the glaucoma, then adjunctive therapy can be added to the therapeutic regime. In any patient in whom topical beta-blockers are not indicated, any of the other topical agents can be initiated as first time therapy. Some relevant findings of the randomized controlled trials are summarized in Ch. Introduction II.
The following pages outline the most frequently used anti-glaucoma medications, and emphasize their mode of action, dosage and side effects. They are to be considered as a general guide, and cannot be all-inclusive.

3.2.1 - THE TARGET INTRAOCULAR PRESSURE (TARGET IOP)

Definition: an estimate of the mean IOP obtained with treatment that is expected to prevent further glaucomatous damage. It is obviously difficult to assess accurately and in advance the IOP level at which further damage may occur in each individual patient and individual eye (see Ch. Introduction II). There is no single IOP level that is safe for every patient. However, it is generally assumed in glaucoma that aiming to achieve at least a 20% reduction from the initial pressure at which damage occurred or in advanced glaucoma to lower the IOP to a level below 18 mmHg at all visits is a useful way to achieve the initial target IOP[14]. In individuals with elevated IOP between 24 mm Hg and 32 mm Hg in one eye and between 21 mm Hg and 32 mm Hg in the other eye, topical ocular hypotensive medication was effective in delaying or preventing the onset of POAG when the IOP was reduced by 20% or an IOP of 24 mm Hg or less was reached[15]. This does not imply however that all patients with borderline or elevated IOP should receive medication. A study comparing treatment vs no treatment in early glaucoma[16-17] showed that lowering the IOP by 25% from baseline determined a 45% decrease in the risk of progression. Patients with POAG with baseline pressures below 30 mm Hg could have a management plan that allows initial observation before treatment to assess the rate of change[16,17] (see Ch. Introduction II). Such an approach is different from the Target Pressure oriented initial approach to POAG and presupposes a monitoring system that allows recognition of change.
The least amount of medication and side effects to achieve the therapeutic response should be a consistent goal (see FC VI).

The target IOP varies according to:

- IOP level before treatment
- The overall risk of IOP-related optic nerve damage, which depends on
    - * average IOP
    - * maximum IOP
    - * fluctuations of IOP

  In case of doubt, consider performing 24 hour or diurnal phasing to identify IOP spikes
- Stage of glaucoma
  The greater the pre-existing glaucoma damage, the lower the target IOP should be.
  In eyes with severe pre-existing damage, any further damage may be functionally important.
- Rate of Progression (RoP) of glaucomatous damage
  Progressive damage is more likely with higher IOP, more severe pre-existing damage and more risk factors.
- Age of patient
- Life expectancy of patient
- Presence of other risk factors
  A lower IOP may be needed if other risk factors are present

Target IOP may need adjustment during the course of the disease

Periodic re-evaluation of individual target IOP considering:

* Efficacy
* Cost vs benefits

If the visual field continues to worsen at a rate that is clinically significant, it may be necessary to aim for a lower target IOP. With the re-evaluation it is important to exclude other risk factors, such as systemic hypotension, poor compliance or IOP spikes[12-22].
Although some benefit can be derived from lowering the IOP even if the target pressure is not reached, the efficacy on the outcome must be assessed carefully in each individual.

Unfortunately one of the limitations of the target IOP approach is that we only know with hindsight whether the target pressure selected initially was adequate or not. In other words a patient must get worse before we verify that the target pressure was inadequate.

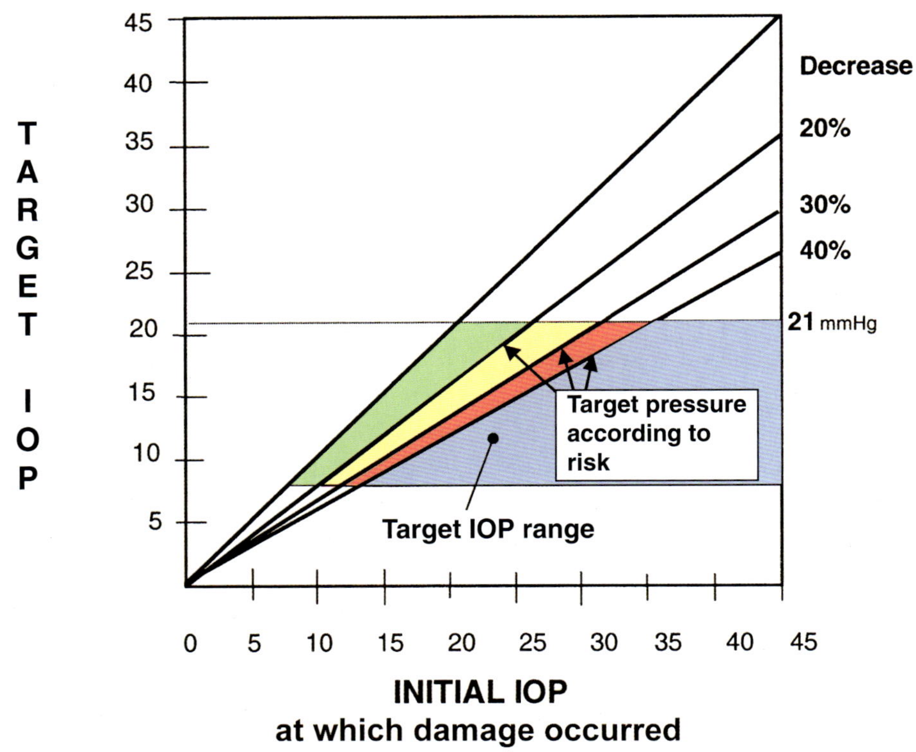

Fig. 3.2.1 - TARGET IOP Diagrammatic evaluation of the desired therapeutic outcome in form of IOP-lowering. The target pressure should be situated within the shaded area. The lower is the initial IOP, the lower will be the Target IOP and viceversa. The percentage of IOP reduction targeted (i.e. 20%, 30%, 40% respectively) depends mainly on the degree of VF damage at diagnosis and on rate of progression (RoP).

3.2.2 - THE QUALITY OF LIFE (QoL)

The quality of life (QoL) is hard to quantify as an outcome measure. For patients however it is one of the most important. Individuals diagnosed with glaucoma can lose quality of life for several reasons[23-32], alone or in combination (see FC I):

a) Diagnosis of glaucoma. Being diagnosed as having a chronic and potentially blinding disease generates worries and anxiety in patients and their families.
b) Functional loss due to the disease
c) Inconvenience of the treatment
d) Side effects of the treatment
e) Cost of the treatment

Each person should be approached by asking their own perceptions on their present status and on their course as well as asked to describe their difficulties with daily tasks (see FC I).

When the disease is not likely to interfere with the QoL, not initiating or witholding treatment is an option to be discussed with the patient.

In order to help our patients to maintain a "healthy" status, we need to focus not only on the treatment of the disease process, but also on the effect of both our diagnosis and treatment on the individual.

Age-Related ganglion cells loss will continue: to reach target IOP is intended to prevent only glaucoma-related functional loss.

REMEMBER:

* Assess each eye individually when deciding the most appropriate therapy.
* It is essential to involve patients as informed partners in decisions regarding the management of their condition.
* The least amount of medication (and consequent inconvenience, costs and side effects) to achieve the therapeutic response should be a consistent goal.
* A therapeutic medical trial on one eye first is useful, although not always logistically feasible.
* Usually there is no need to start treatment until all baseline diagnostic data are collected.
* A single IOP measurement, unless grossly abnormal, is an insufficient parameter upon which solely base the diagnosis and future patient management.

It is important when selecting medical treatment of glaucoma to understand not only the aims of therapy, but also the mode of action, side effects and contraindications of each individual medication.
It is worth remembering that the preservatives contained within topical eye drop preparations may cause inflammatory conjunctival side effects and cytotoxic effects on the ocular surface[33-35]. It is therefore important to consider the use of preservative-free preparations/delivery systems.

Over the past few years there has been a gradual shift in the choice of medical therapy[36-40]. Prostaglandin derivatives/prostamides (such as bimatoprost, latanoprost and travoprost) have in the hands of many ophthalmolgist superceded β-blockers as their first choice. Latanoprost was approved as first-line treatment by EMEA in March 2002 while applications have also been made for bimatoprost and travoprost. The CPMP extended travoprost to first-line treatment in April 2003. There is an ongoing debate in the scientific community regarding the different prostaglandins and prostamides which has not yet been settled.

If the first choice monotherapy alone is not effective on IOP or not tolerated, it is preferrable to switch to any of the other topical agents that can be initiated as monotherapy. If the first choice monotherapy is well tolerated and effective, but not sufficient to reach the target IOP, then adjunctive therapy in the form of any other topical agent can be initiated (see FC VII, VIII and IX).
It is rare nowadays for patients to be maintained on oral carbonic anhydrase inhibitors, because of their adverse systemic side-effects.

INITIAL TREATMENT

<u>First choice treatment</u>:

A drug that a physician prefers to use as initial IOP lowering therapy.

<u>First line treatment:</u>

A drug that has been approved by an official controlling body (i.e. EMEA, CPMP or FDA) for initial IOP lowering therapy.

<u>Therapeutical trial</u>

Where practical, topical treatment is started in one eye at a time.
The differential IOP will give a better idea of the effect, with less influence from diurnal variations.
For some drugs, a cross-over effect to the fellow eye must be taken into account[41-50].

<u>Therapeutic Index</u>

It is the ratio of desired, beneficial effects to adverse effects.

Treatment is considered “effective” on IOP when the observed effect is at least equal to the pubished average effect for the same molecule on a similar population. It must be larger than tonometry errors / variations.

Practical points for topical medical treatment[30,51]

To minimize drainage into the nose or throat, patients should be instructed to use finger pressure exerted on the medial canthus for a minute or two following installation of the eye drop. Excess solution around the eye should be removed with a tissue and any medication on the hands should be rinsed off.

Many studies are available to compare the IOP lowering efficacy and the safety of topical preparations. Published studies vary considerably in population sample, methodology, criteria for definition of the outcome, statistical analysis graphics and overall quality, making very difficult to draw conclusions and comparisons. Meta-analysis is not available for any of the drugs used for glaucoma treatment with the exception of beta blockers. The pre-post graph shown below is a useful tool to show the IOP changes induced by treatment and its use should be encouraged in publications.

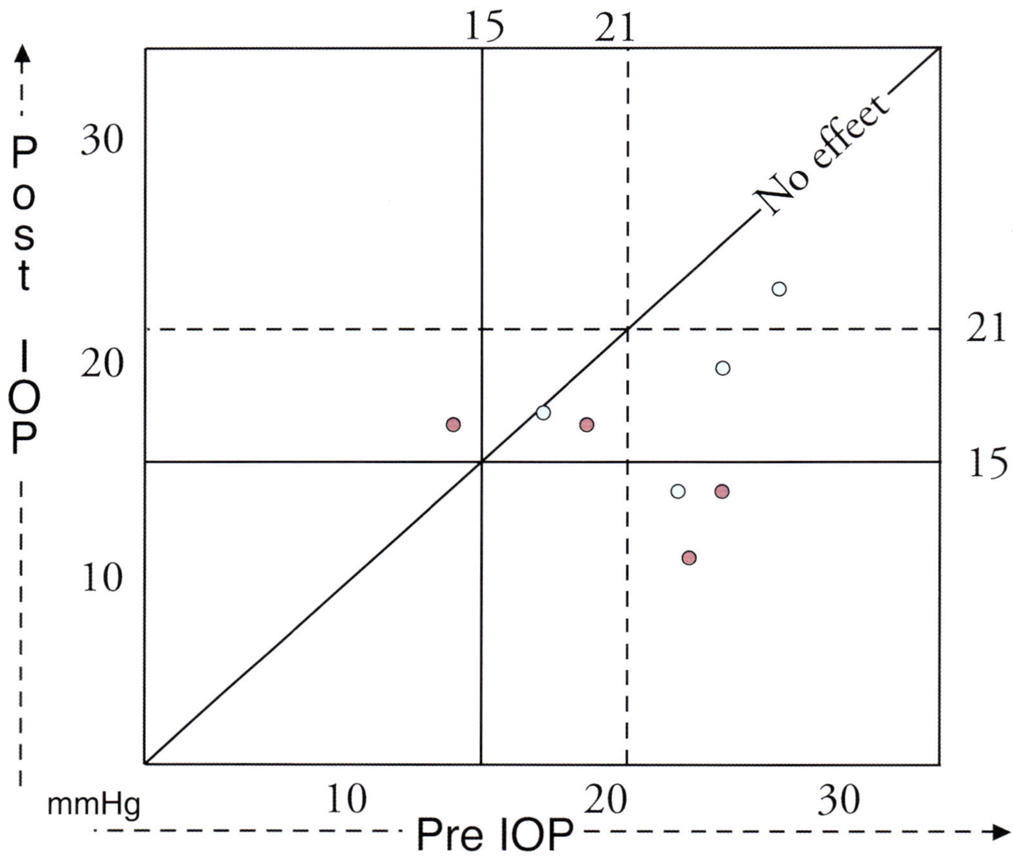

Fig. 3.3 - THE PRE -POST IOP GRAPH
A simple graph can be used to show the IOP lowering effect. Different shapes/colors can be used to show different patient series or different observation times. Vertical and horizontal lines show respectively Pre and Post Treatment IOP levels of interest, here placed as examples at 15 and 21mmHg. Areas of desired effect under the oblique "no effect" line can thus be defined.

The following pages outline the most frequently used anti-glaucoma medications, and emphasize their mode of action, dosage and side effects. They are to be considered as a general guide, and cannot be all-inclusive.

The text does not contain all the drugs, nor all their indications, contraindications and side effects but only the most relevant ones. Before starting each treatment please carefully read the product information sheet.
For each drug category: Action, Dosage and Administration, Indications, Major contraindications, Major side effects, Pregnancy and nursing mothers precautions, Drug interaction, Wash-out are summarized.
When more than one drug is referred to under any heading, these are listed in alphabetical order.

MAIN FEATURES OF SIX FAMILIES OF ANTIGLAUCOMA AGENTS

	ß Blockers	Alpha-2 selective adrenergic agonists (Brimonidine)	Prostaglandin derivatives Prostamides	Topical CAIs	Pilocarpine	Dipivefrin Epinephrine
IOP reduction efficacy	+++ 20-25%	++ to +++ 20-25%	++++ (*) 25-30%	+ to ++ 15-20%	+++ 20-25%	+to++ 15-20%
Cost	+	++	+++	++	+	+
Instillation frequency	1-2 times daily	2-3 times daily	Once daily (*)	2-3 times daily	3-4 times daily	2-3 times daily
Topical tolerability	+++	++	++ to +++	+to+++	++to+++	+++
Topical allergies	+/-	++	+/-	+/-	+/-	++
Preservative free preparations available	Yes	No	No	No	Yes	No
Conjunctival hyperaemia	+/-	+ to ++	+ to ++	-	-	-
Hypertrichosis	-	-	+ to +++	+/-	+/-	++ to +++
Iris darkening	+/-	-	++ to +++	-	-	-
Uveitis	-	-	+ to +++	-	-	-
CME	-	-	+ to +++	-	-	-
Corneal oedema	-	-	-	+/-	-	-
Recurrence HSV keratitis	-	-	+/-	-	-	++
Miosis, browache	-	-	-	+/-	+++	-
Systemic effects:						
Bradyarrhythmias/hypotension	+	-	-	-	-	-
Tachycardia/hypertension	-	-	-	-	-	+
Bronchoconstriction	+++	-	-	-	++	-
Elevated serum lipids	+++	-	-	-	-	-
Increased falls in the elderly	++	-	-	-	-	-
Apnoea in infants	-	++	-	-	-	-
Drowsiness/anergy/fatigue	++	+++	-	-	-	-
Dry mouth	+/-	+ to +++	-	-	-	-

CAIs = carbonic anhydrase inhibitors. CME: Cystoid macular edema
*) Unoprostone: 2 times daily, 20% IOP reduction
Where figures are not used, the scale 0 (minimum) to ++++ (maximun) is used

3.3.1.1 - Category: ADRENERGIC AGONISTS[40-42]

	Generics	Tradenames
Non-selective:	Dipivefrin 0.1%	Propine, Epinal, d-Epifrin, Glaucothil
	Epinephrine 0.25-2.0%	Epinephrine
Alpha-2 selective:	Apraclonidine 0.5-1.0%	Iopidine
	Brimonidine 0.2%	Alphagan
	Clonidine 0.125 -0.5%	Isoglaucon, Catapres, Glaucopres Aruclonin, Clonidophthal

<u>Action</u>

Non-selective:
- Decreases aqueous humor production
- Increases aqueous humor outflow

Alpha-2 selective:

Apraclonidine
- Decreases aqueous humor production
- Maximum effect: 4-5 hours
- Duration of effect: 12 hours
- Reduces IOP 25-39% as monotherapy
- Is additive to timolol
- Additivity to maximum medical therapy

Brimonidine
- Decreases aqueous humor production
- Increases uveoscleral outflow
- Duration of effect: 12h
- Reduces IOP up to 27% as monotherapy
- Selectivity for α_2 vs α_1 adrenoceptors is 1000/1. This selectivity results in no mydriasis and the absence of vasoconstriction.

Clonidine
- Decreases aqueous humor production
- Duration of effect: 6-12 hours
- Little effect on pupillary diameter or accommodation

<u>Dosage and administration</u>

Non-selective:	Dipivefrin 0.1%	2 times daily
	Epinephrine 0.25-2.0%	3 times daily
Alpha-2 selective:	Apraclonidine 0.5-1.0%	2-3 times daily
	Brimonidine 0.2%	2 times daily
	Clonidine 0.125-0.5%	3 times daily

<u>Indications</u>

Non-selective:	Dipivefrin 0.1%	2 times daily Elevation of intraocular pressure in patients where the IOP can be deleterious for the preservation of visual function.
	Epinephrine 0.25-2.0%	3 times daily The same

Alpha-2 selective:	Apraclonidine 0.5%	For temporary chronic dosing as adjunctive treatment on maximally tolerated medical therapy where additional IOP lowering is required (increased risk of allergy with time). The addition of apraclonidine to patients already using two aqueous suppressing drugs (i.e. beta-blocker plus carbonic anhydrase inhibitor) may not provide additional IOP lowering effect.
	Apraclonidine 1.0%	To control or prevent severe elevations in IOP following anterior segment laser procedures.
	Brimonidine 0.2%	Elevation of intraocular pressure in patients where the IOP can be deleterious for the preservation of visual function. Useful as adjunctive treatment or as monotherapy.
	Clonidine 0.125-0.5%	Elevations of intraocular pressure in patients where the IOP can be deleterious for the preservation of visual function.

Major contraindications

Non-selective:	Occludable angles (iridotomy needed) Aphakic patients (macular edema)
Alpha-2 selective:	Oral monoamine oxidase (MAO) inhibitor users Pediatric age

Most frequent side effects

Non-selective:	Follicular conjuctivitis, tachycardia, arrhythmias and arterial hypertension
Alpha-2 selective:	Dry mouth Lid elevation Pupil dilation for apraclonidine No effect on the pupil for brimonidine Allergy (brimonidine up to 15%, apraclonidine up to 36%) Decrease in systolic blood pressure (clonidine) Fatigue, sleepiness (brimonidine), especially in children.

Pregnancy and nursing mothers

Only to be used if the potential benefit justifies the potential risk to the fetus or the infant.

Drug interactions

Possibility of additive or potentiating effect with CNS depressants. Caution is advised in the patients taking tricyclic antidepressant.

Apraclonidine and brimonidine should not be used in small children and patients receiving MAO inhibitors.

Wash-out

The time needed for these compounds to completely lose their action is 1-3 weeks

3.3.1.2 - Category: ADRENERGIC ANTAGONISTS[36,43]

ß-Blockers

	Generics	Tradenames
Beta-1 selective:	Betaxolol 0.5 - 0.25%	Betoptic, Betoptic S, Betoptima
Non-selective:	Befunolol 0.5%	Betaclar
	Levobunolol 0.25, 0.5%	Betagan, Vistagan
	Metipranolol 0.1, 0.3%	Betaman, Beta-ophtiole, Glausyn, Optipranolol, Turoptin
	Timolol 0.1, 0.25, 0.5%	Aquanil, Arutimol, Cusimolol, Nyogel, Optimol, Oftamolol, Timoptic, Timoptic-XE, Timoptol, Timoptol, Timabak, Timogel, Timolabak, Timosine XE, Timosan Depot
With ISA*:	Carteolol 0.5-2.0%	Carteolol 0.5%,1%, 2% Carteol, Carteabak Ocupress, Teoptic, Arteoptic
	Pindolol 2%	Pindoptic

*ISA: Intrinsic Sympathomimetic Activity. The clinical relevance of ISA in glaucoma therapy has not yet been proven.

Action
Decreases intraocular pressure by reduction of the aqueous humor production. Peak effect in 2 hrs.

Dosage and administration
Starting dose is one drop of lowest concentration of solution in the affected eye once or twice a day. If the clinical response is not adequate, the dosage may be increased to one drop of a higher concentration. Nyogel, Timolol in gel-rite (Timoptic-XE, Timacar Depot, Timoptol XE, and Timosan Depot) is given once daily.
No dose response curves for the different beta-blocker treatments have been established. The lowest concentration that would give the expected clinical effect should be used to avoid side defects. Dosing more than twice daily will not give any further pressure lowering effect.
Minimal extra effect with dipivefrine. No extra effect with adrenaline (epinephrine). Additive effect with most other IOP-lowering agents.
Preservativa-free preparations are available and may be considered.

Indications
Elevation of intraocular pressure in patients where the IOP can be deleterious for the preservation of visual function. Beta-1 selective adrenergic antagonist despite lowering IOP less than non selective, protect visual field as well as non selective ones.

Major Contraindications
Non-selective: Asthma, history of obstructive pulmonary disease, sinus bradycardia (< 60 beats/min), heart block, or cardiac failure
Beta-1 selective: Relative contraindication in asthma, history of obstructive pulmonary disease, sinus bradycardia (< 60 beats/min), heart block, or cardiac failure.

Major side effects
Non-selective: *Systemic*: Bradycardia, arrhythmia, heart failure, syncope, bronchospasm, and airways obstruction. Distal edema, hypotension. Depression. Hypoglycemia may be masked in insulin dependent diabetes mellitus. Beta-blocking agents have been associated with nocturnal hypotension, which may be a risk factor in progression of glaucomatous optic nerve damage[52].
Ocular (uncommon): Epithelial keratopathy, slight reduction in corneal sensitivity.

Beta-1 selective: Better tolerated in most patients sensitive to non-selective agents.

Pregnancy and nursing mothers

Only to be used if the potential benefit justifies the potential risk to the fetus or the infant.

Drug interactions

Oral or intravenous calcium antagonists: caution should be used in the co-administration of beta-adrenergic blocking agents and oral or intravenous calcium antagonists, because of possible atrioventricular conduction disturbances, left ventricular failure, and hypotension.

Digitalis and calcium antagonists: the concomitant use of beta-adrenergic blocking agents with digitalis may have additive effects in prolonging conduction time.

Catecholamine-depleting drugs: possible additive effects and the production of hypotension and/or marked bradycardia.

Wash-out

The time needed for beta blockers to completely lose their activity is 2-5 weeks.

3.3.1.3 - Category: CARBONIC ANHYDRASE INHIBITORS[46]

	Generics	Tradenames
Topical:	Brinzolamide 1% Dorzolamide 2%	Azopt Trusopt
Systemic:	Acetazolamide	Diamox, Diamox Sequels, Diamox Retard
	Dichlorphenamide Methazolamide	Antidrasi, Daranide, Glaumid, Oralcon Neptazane

Action

Topical: Carbonic anhydrase inhibitor. Reduces aqueous formation resulting in lowered IOP.
Systemic: Carbonic anhydrase inhibitor. Reduces aqueous formation resulting in lowered IOP.

Dosage and administration

Topical:	Dorzolamide 2%	Monotherapy: three times daily. As adjunctive therapy with topical betablocker: two times daily
	Brinzolamide 1%	Monotherapy: two - three times daily As adjunctive therapy with topical betablocker: two times daily
Systemic:	Acetazolamide	250 mg tablets (given QID as full dose) 500 mg slow- release capsule (given BID as full dose)
	Dichlorphenamide	50 mg 1-3 times daily
	Methazolamide	50-100 mg 2-3 times daily

Indications

Topical: Elevations of intraocular pressure in patients where the IOP can be deleterious for the preservation of visual function.

Systemic: When topical medications not effective or feasible. When long-term systemic CAI are needed, glaucoma surgery should be considered.

Major contraindications

Topical: Hypersensitivity to any component of the product

Systemic: Contraindicated in situations in which sodium and/or potassium blood levels are depressed, in cases of kidney and liver disease or dysfunction, in suprarenal gland failure, and in hyperchloremic acidosis.

Precautions

Topical: For the treatment of acute angle-closure glaucoma attack with corneal edema and inflamed conjunctiva, systemic CAI treatment is preferable.
In patients with low corneal endothelial cell count, there is increased risk of corneal edema.
Since no data on patients with severe renal impairment (CrCl < 30 mL/ml) are available, they should not be used in such patients. The concomitant use of topical and oral carbonic anhydrase inhibitors is not additive and not recommended.
These compounds are sulfonamides; the same kind of adverse reactions that are attributable to any sulfonamide may occur.

Systemic: Increasing the dose may increase the incidence of drowsiness and /or paresthesia. Adverse reaction common to all sulfonamide derivatives may occur like anaphylaxis, fever rash (erythema multiforme), Stevens-Johnson syndrome, bone marrow depression, thrombocytopenic purpura, hemolytic anemia, leukopenia, pancytopenia and agranulocytosis. Some of the above can be irreversible and lethal. If the patient is on another diuretic orally periodic monitoring of serum electrolytes is indicated.

Major side effects

Topical: Ocular burning, stinging, bitter taste, superficial punctate keratitis, blurred vision, tearing, headache, urticaria, angioedema, pruritus, asthenia, dizziness, paresthesia and transient myopia.

Systemic: Paresthesias, hearing dysfunction, tinnitus, loss of appetite, taste alteration, gastrointestinal disturbances such as nausea, vomiting and diarrhoea. Depression, decreased libido, gastrointestinal symptoms, kidney stones, blood dyscrasias. Metabolic acidosis and electrolyte imbalance may occur.

Adverse reaction common to all sulfonamide derivatives may occur like anaphylaxis, fever rash (erythema multiforme), Steven-Johnson syndrome, bone marrow depression, thrombocytopenic purpura, hemolytic anemia, leukopenia, pancytopenia and agranulocytosis.

Pregnancy and nursing mothers

Topical: Only to be used if the potential benefit justifies the potential risk to the fetus or the infant.

Systemic: Only to be used if the potential benefit justifies the potential risk to the fetus or the infant.(Teratogenic effect seen from high doses of systemic CAIs in some animal species). Women of childbearing age should be warned of possible teratogenic effect.

Drug interactions

Topical: Specific drug interaction studies have not yet been performed

Systemic: Should be used with caution in patients on steroid therapy because of the potential for developing hypokalemia.

Wash-out

The time needed to completely lose their activity:

Topical CAI	1 week
Systemic CAI	3 days

3.3.1.4 - Category: PARASYMPATHOMIMETICS (CHOLINERGIC DRUGS)[44,45]

	Generics	Tradenames
Direct-acting:	Pilocarpine 0.5-4%	E-pilo, Isopto Carpine, Pilagan, Pilocar, Pilogel, Pilomann, Pilopine, Pilopine HS Gel, Pilostat, Spersacarpine, Isopto Carpine
	Aceclidine 2%	Glaucostat Glaucostate, Glaunorm
	Carbachol 0.75-3%	Isopto Carbachol, Karbakolin Isopto
	Acetylcholine 1%	Miochol
Indirect-acting:	Demecarium bromide 0.125, 0.25%	Humorsol, Tosmilen
	Ecothiophate iodide 0.03-0.25%	Phospholine Iodide, Echodide
	Physostigmine	Eserine
Combinations:	Pilocarpine + Physostigmine	Piloeserine
	Carbachol 0.75% + Pilocarpine 2% +HCl Procaine 2%	Mios

Action

Increase in facility of outflow of aqueous humor.
Direct action on longitudinal ciliary muscle.

Dosage and administration

Direct-acting:

Pilocarpine 1-4%	Lowers IOP after 1 hr, lasts 6-7 hrs; usually given QID or TID in solutions with hydrophilic polymers.
Pilocarpine gel	Once daily at bedtime.
Ocuserts 20 or 40 µg/hr	Usually once weekly
Carbachol 0.75%, 1.5%, 2.25%, and 3%	Three times daily.
Acetylcholine 1:100 solution	For intracameral use during surgery
Aceclidine 2%	BID (induces less accommodative spasm, a smaller increase in lens thickness and a lower reduction of the chamber depth compared to pilocarpine).

Indirect-acting:

Demecarium bromide 0.125 and 0.25%	Twice a day, at bedtime and in the morning.
Ecothiophate iodide 0.03-0.25%	Once or twice a day, at bedtime and in the morning.

Indications

Direct-acting: Elevation of intraocular pressure in patients where the IOP can be deleterious for the preservation of visual function.

Indirect-acting: POAG in aphakia / pseudophakia where surgery is refused or not feasible, in cases that are not con trolled on other less potent agents.
These cases may respond satisfactory to ecothiophate iodide 0.03% or demecarium bromide 0.125% twice a day.

Major contraindications

Direct-acting: Age < 40 yrs, cataract, uveitis and neovascular glaucoma. Assess possible worsening of pupillary block in each case of angle-closure glaucoma.

Indirect-acting: Active uveitis.

Precautions

Direct-acting: Axial myopia, history of retinal detachment or rhegmatogenous retinal lesions.

Indirect-acting: Should be used with extreme caution in patients with marked vagotonia, bronchial asthma, spastic gastrointestinal disturbances, peptic ulcer, pronounced bradycardia and hypotension, recent myocardial infarction, epilepsy and Parkinsonism. Priory history of retinal detachment or rhegmatogenous retinal lesions.

General anesthesia with curarization.

Major side effects

Direct-acting: Systemic: Intestinal cramps, branchospasm.

Ocular: Miosis, pseudomyopia (up to 8D), browache, retinal detachment, ciliary spasm, increased pupillary block.

Indirect-acting: Systemic: Cardiac irregularities, intestinal cramps.

Ocular: Stinging, burning, lacrimation, browache, pseudomyopia, retinal detachment, conjunctival thickening, increased pupillary block, iris cysts, cataract.

Pregnancy and nursing mothers

Direct-acting: Only to be used if the potential benefit justifies the potential risk to the fetus or the infant.

Indirect-acting: Contraindicated

Drug interactions

Direct-acting: A competitive interaction on outflow with prostaglandins is assumed, since contraction of the ciliary muscle reduces the uveoscleral space.

Indirect-acting: Patients undergoing systemic anticholinesterase treatment should be warned of the possible additive effects of the indirect-acting parasympathomimetics. General anesthesia with muscle relaxants.

Wash-out

The time needed to completely lose their activity: *Direct acting*: 3 days

Indirect acting: several weeks. Some are irreversible.

3.3.1.5 - Category: PROSTAGLANDIN DERIVATIVES AND PROSTAMIDES[47,53-73]

	Generics	Tradenames
Topical:	Bimatoprost 0.03%	Lumigan
	Latanoprost 0.005%	Xalatan
	Travoprost 0.004%	Travatan
	Unoprostone 0.12%, 0.15%	Rescula

	Lumigan®	Xalatan®	Travatan®	Rescula®
Active ingredient*	*Bimatoprost*	*Latanoprost*	*Travoprost*	*Unoprostone*
Category	*Prostamide*	*Prostaglandin*	*Prostaglandin*	*Docosanoid*
Formulation	*0.03%*	*0.005%*	*0.004%*	*0.12%, 0.15%*
Preservative	*BAC 0.05 mg/ml*	*BAC 0.2 mg/ml*	*BAC 0.15 mg/ml*	*BAC 0.1 mg/ml*
	0.005%	*0.002%*	*0.015%*	*0.01%*
Dosage	*Once daily*	*Once daily*	*Once daily*	*Twice daily*
*in alphabetic order				

Action

For bimatoprost, latanoprost and travoprost the most evident action is the increase of the uveo-scleral outflow, reducing IOP 20% - 35%.

The IOP lowering effect of unoprostone is up to 18% from baseline. Unoprostone 0.12% has been available in Japan since 1994.

Pressure lowering effect:[53-61]

Bimatoprost	7-8 mmHg	(baseline 26 mmHg)
Latanoprost	6-8 mmHg	(baseline 24-25 mmHg)
Travoprost	7-8 mmHg	(baseline 25-27 mmHg)
Unoprostone	3-4 mmHg	(baseline 24-25 mmHg)

Reduction of the intraocular pressure starts approximately 2-4 hours after the first administration with peak effect reached within approximately 8 to 12 hours. Maximum IOP lowering is often achieved 3 to 5 weeks from commencement of treatment

Dosage and administration

Bimatoprost 0.03%, latanoprost 0.005% or travoprost 0.004% solution: once daily, preferably in the evening.
Unoprostone 0.12% and 0.15% BID.

Indications

Latanoprost has received European (EMEA) and FDA approval as first line drug for reducing intraocular pressure (IOP) in patients with open-angle glaucoma or ocular hypertension. A similar application as first-line treatment for bimatoprost and travoprost have now also been made to the European regulatory agencies. The CPMP extended the indication for travoprost to first-line treatment in April 2003.

There are only few published clinical trials with bimatoprost, latanoprost, travoprost and unoprostone in treating angle-closure glaucoma, inflammatory or neovascular glaucoma. Most of the large clinical trials of unoprostone are on the Japanese population.

The prostaglandin analogues and prostamides (bimatoprost, latanoprost, travoprost and unoprostone) appear to be effective, well-tolerated agents for the reduction of intraocular pressure (IOP) in patients with primary open-angle glaucoma and ocular hypertension; most of the long-term data are published on latanoprost.

This drug class offers potential as first choice drugs or an alternative for patients who do not achieve control the target IOP with another topical antiglaucoma agent or for those with a contraindication to initial therapy with beta-adrenergic antagonists. Based on preliminary clinical data, bimatoprost, latanoprost, and travoprost appear to be at least as effective on IOP as timolol, while the effectiveness of unoprostone is similar or slightly less.

Prostaglandin analogues/prostamide may be used in conjunction with other antiglaucoma medications, although further studies must establish the optimal combinations. Whether clinical experience will yield outcomes in favour of one of these products remains to be determined. Patients should be educated on associated adverse events especially pigmentation of the iris and eyelashes.

Major contraindications

Known hypersensitivity to bimatoprost / latanoprost / travoprost / unoprostone, benzalkonium chloride, or any other product ingredient.

Patients should not administer these drugs while wearing contact lenses, but contact lenses can be reinserted 15 minutes following administration of the drugs.

Precautions

Cystoid macular edema in aphakes/pseudophakes has been reported in few cases, most occurring in aphakic patients, in pseudophakic patients with a posterior lens capsule rupture, or in patients with known risk factors for macular edema[69,70].

Bimatoprost, latanoprost, travoprost and unoprostone should be used with caution in these patients although con current administration of nonsteroidal anti-inflammatory agents, such as diclofenac, might decrease this side effect

Unilateral treatment may cause a difference in iris colour and in length, thickness, pigmentation, and number of lashes between the eyes.

Patients with uveitis.

Side effects

Local:

Conjunctival hyperemia (Bimatoprost up to 44.7%[53], Latanoprost up to 27.6%[55], Travoprost up to 49.5%[55], Unoprostone up to 9%[61]), burning and stinging, foreign body sensation and itching. Hyperemia is often transient and usually mild, without associated symptoms.

Eyelash changes (increased length, thickness, pigmentation, and number of lashes), reversible after cessation of medication[52-58,65].

Increased iris pigmentation, especially seen in patients with green-brown, blue/gray-brown or yellow-brown irides. The long-term effects on the iris or other parts of the eye are currently unknown. This effect is to be considered permanent[62-64]. Unoprostone is less likely to change iris color.

Cystoid macular edema in aphakes/pseudophakes has been reported in few cases, most occurring in aphakic patients, in pseudophakic patients with a posterior lens capsule rupture, or in patients with known risk factors for macular edema[69,70].

Reactivation of herpes keratitis[66,67].

Anterior uveitis[68].

Systemic:

The following events have been identified during postmarketing use of prostaglandin analogues in clinical practice. Because they are reported voluntarily from a population of unknown size, estimates of frequency cannot be made.The events include: dyspnea, asthma and exacerbation of asthma.

Prostaglandin derivatives and prostamides appears to have very few systemic side effects in comparison with β blockers and selective $\alpha 2$ agonists[71-73].

Pregnancy and nursing mothers

There are no adequate and well controlled studies in pregnant women. Only to be used during pregnancy if potential benefit justifies the potential risk to the fetus.

It is not known whether the drugs or their metabolites are excreted in human milk.

Drug interactions
Precipitation occurs when thiomerosal-containing eye drops are mixed with bimatoprost, latanoprost or travoprost. Administer such drugs at least 5 minutes apart.

Wash-out
The time needed for topical prostaglandins to lose their action completely is 4-6 weeks.

There is some ongoing discussion regarding differences between prostaglandin derivatives and prostamides, which has not been settled yet in the scientific comunity.
Patients may respond differently to these agents[51].
The EMEA has approved the use of the term prostamide.

3.3.1.6 - OSMOTICS

Hyperosmotics are the most effective agents. The patients must be evaluated for heart or kidney disease because hyperosmotics increase blood volume which increases the load on the heart. They may alter glucose blood levels and should be given to diabetics only with great caution and monitoring.

- Glycerol 1.0 - 1.5 g/Kg orally
- Mannitol 1.0 - 1.5 g/Kg intravenously

3.3.2 - COMBINED DRUGS PREPARATIONS

Rational for drug combinations.
Antiglaucoma eye drops can be combined with each other, as well as added to laser and surgical treatments.
Drugs which belong to the same pharmacological group should not be used in combination (e.g. do not combine two different beta-blockers).

- When available, combined drugs preparations are generally preferrable to two separate instillations of the same agents; this is due to improved compliance and positive influence on dosing schedule and quality of life.
- To use more than two drugs in combination is not recommended in most patients (see Ch. 3.4).
- The additional drug(s) should be used only if needed to obtain the aimed-for target IOP.
- The effect of drug combinations is only measured in terms of IOP reduction.
- Assuming equal IOP effects, no drug combination is yet known to be preferable in terms of ONH or VF preservation.
- If the first choice treatment has no effect, or tachyphylaxis occurs, change the initial therapy rather than adding a further drug.
- Increasing the recommended dosage will not result in increased IOP lowering and will only cause more side effects.

DRUG COMBINATIONS - ADDITIVE EFFECT

CURRENT DRUG	ADDITIONAL DURG				
	α2 agonists	β-blockers	Topical CAIs	Cholinergic	Prostaglandin/Prostamides
α2 agonists		+	+	+	+
β-blockers	+		+	+	+
Topical CAIs	+	+		+	+
Cholinergic	+	+	+		+/-
Prostaglandins/ prostamides	+	+	+	+/-	

COMBINATION THERAPY

Starting*	Additional*	Remarks
α2-agonists	β-blockers	
	topical CAI	Good additive IOP - lowering effect
	prostaglandis	
	prostamides	
	sympathomimetics	Additional IOP lowering effect is relatively poor
β-blockers	α_2-agonist	Good additive IOP - lowering effect
	topical CAIs	Good additive IOP - lowering effect Available in combined preparation
	prostaglandins	Good additive IOP - lowering effect Available in combined preparation
	prostamides	Good additive IOP - lowering effect
	sympathomimetics	
Topical CAIs	α_2-agonists	
	β-blockers	Available in combined preparation
	prostaglandins	
	prostamides	
	sympathomimetics	Additional IOP lowering effect is relatively poor
Cholinergic	α_2-agonists	
	β-blockers	Available in combined preparation
	topical CAIs	
Prostaglandin	α_2-agonists	
	β-blockers	Available in combined preparation
	topical CAI	
	sympathomimetics	
Prostamides	α_2-agonists	
	β-blockers	
	topical CAI	
	sympathomimetics	

* these columns are listed in alphabetic order

3.3.2.1 - Category: *ADRENERGIC ANTAGONISTS AND PARASYMPATHOMIMETICS*

ß-Blockers & Pilocarpine

Generics	Tradenames
Metipranolol 0.1% and pilocarpine 2%	Ripix, Normoglaucon
Timolol 0.5% and pilocarpine 1% to 4%	Timpilo, Fotil ,Equiton, Timicon.
Carteolol 2% and Pilocarpine	Carpilo

Action
Decreased intraocular pressure by reduction of the aqueous humor production.
Increase a facility of outflow of aqueous humor. Direct action on longitudinal ciliary muscle.
Peak effect in 2 hrs.

Dosage and administration
Starting dose is one drop of lowest concentration of solution in the affected eye twice a day. If the clinical response is not adequate, the dosage may be increased to one drop of a higher concentration. Dosing more than twice daily will not give any further pressure lowering effect.

Indications
Elevations of intraocular pressure in patients where the IOP can be deleterious for the preservation of visual function, where the target IOP is not obtained with less potent agents.

Major Contraindications
Asthma, history of obstructive pulmonary disease, sinus bradycardia (< 60 beats/min), heart block, or cardiac failure. Relative contraindication in history of obstructive pulmonary disease,
Young age < 40 yrs old, cataract, uveitis and neovascular glaucoma. Assess worsening of pupillary block in angle-closure glaucomas.

Precautions
Extreme caution in patients with marked vagotonia, bronchial asthma, spastic gastrointestinal disturbances, peptic ulcer, pronounced bradycardia and hyotension, recent myocardial infarction, epilepsy and Parkinsonism. Prior history of retinal detachment or rhegmatogenous retinal lesions.

Major side effects
Systemic: Bradycardia, arrhythmia, heart failure, syncope, bronchospasm, and airways obstruction. Peripheral edema, hypotension. Depression. Hypoglycemia may be masked in insulin dependent diabetes mellitus. Intestinal cramps.
Ocular: Epithelial keratopathy, slight reduction in corneal sensitivity. Miosis, pseudomyopia, browache, retinal detachment, ciliary spasm, increased pupillary block.

Pregnancy and nursing mothers
Only to be used if the potential benefit justifies the potential risk to the fetus or the infant.

Drug interactions
Caution should be used in the co-administration of beta-adrenergic blocking agents and oral or intravenous calcium antagonists, because of possible atrioventricular conduction disturbances, left ventricular failure, and hypotension.
Digitalis and calcium antagonists: the concomitant use of beta-adrenergic blocking agents with digitalis and calcium antagonists may have additive effects in prolonging conduction time.
A competitive dualism on outflow with prostaglandins is assumed, since parasympathomimetics induce contraction of the ciliary muscle which reduces the uveoscleral space.

Wash-out
The time needed for beta blockers to lose their activity completely is 2-4 weeks; for pilocarpine is 1-3 days.

3.3.2.2 - Category: ADRENERGIC ANTAGONISTS AND TOPICAL C.A.I.[74-75]

ß-Blockers & topical CAI

Generics	Tradenames
Timolol 0.5% and dorzolamide 2%	Cosopt

Action

Decreases intraocular pressure by reduction of the aqueous humor production. Peak effect in 2 hrs.

Dosage and administration

Starting dose is one drop in the affected eye twice a day. Dosing more than twice daily will not give any further pressure lowering effect.

Additive effect with pilocarpine. Minimal extra effect with dipivefrine. No extra effect with adrenaline (epinephrine).

Indications

Elevations of intraocular pressure in patients where the IOP can be deleterious for the preservation of visual function.

Major Contraindications

Asthma, history of obstructive pulmonary disease, sinus bradycardia (< 60 beats/min), heart block, or cardiac failure, severe renal impairment (CrCl < 30 ml/min) or hyperchloremic acidosis, hypersensitivity to any component of the product. Relative contraindication in history of obstructive pulmonary disease.

Major side effects

Systemic: Bradycardia, arrhythmia, heart failure, syncope, bronchospasm, and airways obstruction. Peripheral edema, hypotension. Depression. Hypoglycemia may be masked in insulin dependent diabetes mellitus.

Ocular (uncommon): Epithelial keratopathy, slight reduction in corneal sensitivity.

Pregnancy and nursing mothers

Only to be used if the potential benefit justifies the potential risk to the fetus or the infant.

Drug interactions

Caution should be used in the co-administration of beta-adrenergic blocking agents and oral or intravenous calcium antagonists, because of possible atrioventricular conduction disturbances, left ventricular failure, and hypotension.

Digitalis and calcium antagonists: the concomitant use of beta-adrenergic blocking agents with digitalis and calcium antagonists may have additive effects in prolonging conduction time.

Catecholamine-depleting drugs: because of possible additive effects and the production of hypotension and/or marked bradycardia.

Wash-out

The time needed to lose their activity completely is 2-4 weeks.

3.3.2.3 - Category: PROSTAGLANDINS AND ADRENERGIC ANTAGONISTS

Prostaglandin & ß-Blocker

Generics	Tradenames
Latanoprost 0.005% and Timolol 0.5%	Xalcom, Xalacom

Action

In latanoprost the most evident action is the increase of the uveo-scleral outflow, reducing IOP 20% - 35%. Timolol decreases intraocular pressure by reduction of the aqueous humor production. Peak effect in 2 hrs. for timolol and 8-12 hours for latanoprost.

Dosage and administration

Starting dose is one drop in the morning.

Indications

Elevation of intraocular pressure in patients where the IOP can be deleterious for the preservation of visual function in spite of medical glaucoma monotherapy.

Major Contraindications

Non-selective β-blockers: Asthma, history of obstructive pulmonary disease, sinus bradycardia (< 60 beats/min), heart block, or cardiac failure

Known hypersensitivity to latanoprost, timolol, benzalkonium chloride, or any other product ingredient.

Patients should not administer these drugs while wearing contact lenses, but contact lenses can be reinserted 15 minutes following administration of the drugs.

Major side effects

Systemic: Bradycardia, arrhythmia, heart failure, syncope, bronchospasm, and airways obstruction. Distal edema, hypotension. Depression. Hypoglycemia may be masked in insulin dependent diabetes mellitus. Beta-blocking agents are associated with nocturnal hypotension, which may be a risk factor in progression of glaucomatous optic nerve damage.

Ocular: Conjunctival hyperemia, burning and stinging, foreign body sensation and itching.
Eyelash changes (increased length, thickness, pigmentation, and number of lashes).
Increased iris pigmentation in patients treated with melanocytes is increased. Especially seen in patients with green-brown, blue/gray-brown or yellow-brown irides. The long-term effects on the melanocytes and the consequences of potential injury to the melanocytes and /or deposition of pigment granules to other areas of the eye are currently unknown. The effect may be permanent.

Cystoid macular edema in aphakes/pseudophakes has been reported in few cases, most occurring in aphakic patients, in pseudophakic patients with a posterior lens capsule rupture, or in patients with known risk factors for macular edema.

Epithelial keratopathy, slight reduction in corneal sensitivity.
Reactivation of herpes keratitis.
Anterior uveitis.

Precautions

Cystoid macular edema in aphakes/pseudophakes has been reported in few cases, most occurring in aphakic patients, in pseudophakic patients with a posterior lens capsule rupture, or in patients with known risk factors for macular edema.

Unilateral treatment may cause a difference in iris colour between the eyes.

Patients with uveitis.

Pregnancy and nursing mothers

Only to be used if the potential benefit justifies the potential risk to the fetus or the infant.

Drug interactions

Oral or intravenous calcium antagonists: caution should be used in the co-administration of beta-adrenergic blocking agents and oral or intravenous calcium antagonists, because of possible atrioventricular conduction disturbances, left ventricular failure, and hypotension.

Digitalis and calcium antagonists: the concomitant use of beta-adrenergic blocking agents with digitalis may have additive effects in prolonging conduction time.

Catecholamine-depleting drugs: possible additive effects and the production of hypotension and/or marked bradycardia.

Wash-out

The time needed for beta blockers & latanoprost to lose their activity completely is 2-5 weeks.

THE WASH-OUT TIME NEEDED FOR A TOPICALLY ADMINISTERED DRUG TO COMPLETELY LOSE ITS EFFECT VARIES GREATLY

Betablockers	2-5 weeks
Sympathomimetics	2 weeks
Direct acting miotics	1-3 days
Indirect-acting miotics	1 month-permanent
Topical CAI	1 week
Oral CAI	1 week
Prostaglandins/ Prostamides	4-6 weeks

Since glaucoma is a long-standing, progressive disease, which frequently requires topical medication and regular follow-up appointments, a patient's continuous co-operation is essential for successful management.
Compliance with glaucoma medications is considerably less than presumed by doctors and many patients fail to attend follow-up appointments[26-30]. Non-compliance is likely to have an important role in the progression to blindness from glaucoma[77]. Glaucoma patients are frequently old and may have diminished cognitive abilities, poor hearing and other ailments which, like arthritis, may reduce their ability to actually administer medication.
Drug interactions and diminished drug tolerance must be taken into consideration. Consultation with other medical practitioners involved in the patient's care may be necessary[23,75].
Compliance issues must be taken into account when the type of treatment is selected.

Poor compliance is summarized as follows:

1. Failure to instill eye drops (including ineffective technique of self-administration)
2. Excessive use of eye drops (extra drops may cause systemic side effects)
3. Self-administration of non-prescribed eye drops
4. Improper timing of eye drops and eye drop administration for wrong reasons (a more frequent problem if nume rous drops are to be instilled and after changes in the patient's topical medication regimen)

How can compliance be improved?

1. Make the patient an active and informed participant in his/her management. Glaucoma itself and the mechanism of the medication prescribed have to be explained. In addition, patients must be informed about the symptoms of potential side effects. Written and audio-visual information can be added to verbal education. If necessary, com munication with the patient's family often helps to improve compliance.
2. The number, concentration of drug and frequency should be kept to a minimum. Ocular irritation may be decreased by reducing the number of preserved eye drops[33-35].
3. Inconvenience caused by the medication has to be minimised, and the times of the eye drop instillation should be linked to landmarks of the patient's daily routine.
4. The patient should be taught how to instill eye drops correctly (correct technique of instillation, lid closure, punctal occlusion, use of instillation frames, time interval between administration of different drops etc). This knowledge is to be checked in practice. Ancillary medical staff can significantly help to accomplish this work.

3.5 - LASER SURGERY

3.5.1 - LASER IRIDOTOMY[76]

Indication

Clinically relevant pupillary block.

Preoperative preparation

- Pilocarpine 2% or 4% single instillation (unfolds the iris, reduces iris thickness, fascilitates perforation)
- Prevention of IOP spikes
  Oral or intravenous acetazolamide
  Topical apraclonidine 1%
  One hour prior to the procedure and immediately afterwards, diminishes the frequency and magnitude of the acute postoperative IOP spikes and decreases bleeding due to the vasoconstrictor effect.
  Remember to check for known drug intolerance or other systemic contraindications.
- Topical anaesthesia
- Topical glycercerine, intravenous mannitol or oral hyperosmotic agents to be considered if the cornea is oedema tous

Procedure

A laser iridotomy contact lens is needed to keep the lids open, stabilize the eye, focus the laser beam and act as a heat sink, while providing additional magnification.

<u>Lenses</u>

- Abraham (+66 dioptres)
- Wise (+103 dioptres)
- CGI © LASAG CH

<u>Iridotomy site</u>

- superior quadrants of the iris covered by the upper lid (to prevent monocular diplopia)
- avoid the 3 o`clock and 9 o`clock positions to lessen discomfort and reduce the risk of hitting the iris vessels
- avoid visible vessels
- as far peripherally as possible within the arcus senilis
- choose a thin looking area or an iris crypt
- electively superonasal to reduce the likelihood of a macular injury when using the Argon laser

<u>Laser parameters</u>

Nd:YAG Laser Iridotomy

Power:	1-6 mJ
Spot size:	50-70 µm (constant for each laser model)
Pulses per burst:	1-3

Focus the beam within the iris stroma rather than on the surface of the iris

Lens capsule damage is possible above 2 mJ energy. Use the least amount of energy that is effective. With most lasers it is unlikely that more than 5 mJ per pulse will be needed.

Argon Laser Iridotomy

When no Nd:YAG laser is available, the Argon laser may be used.
There is no single group of laser parameters for all types of iris and for all surgeons
The laser parameters need to be adjusted intraoperatively

Preparatory stretch burns:		Penetration burns:	
Spot size:	200-500 µm	Spot Size:	50 µm
Exposure time:	0.2-0.6 seconds	Exposure time:	0.2 seconds
Power:	200-600 mW	Power:	800-1000 mW

For pale blue or hazel irides, the following parameters are suggested:

First step: to obtain a gas bubble	Spot Size	50 µm
	Exposure time	0.5 seconds
	Power:	1500 mW
Second step: penetration through the gas bubble	Spot Size	50 µm
	Exposure time	0.05 seconds
	Power	1000 mW

For thick, dark brown irides:

Chipping technique	Spot Size	50 µm
	Exposure time	0.02 seconds
	Power	1500-2500 mW

The purpose of the procedure is to obtain a full thickness hole of sufficient diameter to resolve the pupillary block. Perforation is assumed when pigment, mixed with aqueous, flows into the anterior chamber. The iris usually falls back and the peripheral anterior chamber deepens. Patency must be confirmed by direct visualization of the lens through the iridotomy. Transillumination through the pupil or the iridotomy is not a reliable indicator of success. The optimal size of the iridotomy is 100 to 500 µm.

Complications:

Temporary blurring of vision
Corneal epithelial and/or endothelial burns with Argon
Intraoperative bleeding, usually controlled by a gentle pressure applied to the eye with the contact lens
Transient elevation of the IOP
Postoperative inflammation
Posterior synechiae
Late closure of the iridotomy
Localized lens opacities
Endothelial damage
Rare complications include retinal damage, cystoid macular edema, sterile hypopion, malignant glaucoma.

Post-operative management:

Check the IOP after 1-3 hours, and again after 24-48 hours. When this is not possible, give prophylactic treatment to avoid IOP spikes
Topical corticosteroids for 4-7 days
Repeat gonioscopy
Pupillary dilatation to break posterior synechiae
Verify the patency of the peripheral iridotomy

3.5.2 - LASER TRABECULOPLASTY[77-89]

Indications:

POAG, exfoliative and pigmentary glaucoma when IOP is not satisfactorily controlled with medications, where the latter are contraindicated, or where compliance is a problem, such as in the elderly.

Should initial medical therapy fail to control the patient's glaucoma, ALT could be offered for patients with heavily pigmented trabecular meshwork and for those patients who are infirm, elderly, or have a short life expectancy.

Preoperative preparation:

- prevention of IOP spikes: topical apraclonidine 1% and/or oral acetazolamide one hour prior to the procedure and immediately afterwards
- topical anaesthesia

Procedure:

Argon laser (Green or Blue/Green)
Diode laser

Lenses:

- Goldmann type gonioscopy lens
- Ritch trabeculoplasty lens©
- CGA© Lasag

- Identify angle landmarks
- Laser burns placed between the anterior pigmented trabecular meshwork and the non-pigmented trabecular meshwork ie mid to anterior third of the trabecular meshwork over 180 or 360 degrees.

If necessary, repeat 2 weeks later over the other 180 degrees if only half circumference was initially treated.
When electing to perform two sessions of 180 degrees, make sure not to repeat the treatment in the same quadrant.

Laser parameters:

Spot Size:	50 µm
Exposure time:	0.1 seconds
Power:	500-1200 mW according to the reaction on the trabecular meshwork
Optimal reaction:	transient blanching or small gas bubble formation

Complications:

Transient decrease in visual acuity due to gonioscopy contact fluid, inflammation, significant IOP elevation
Transient iritis
Early and transient IOP elevations
Visual field loss as a consequence of IOP spikes
Peripheral anterior synechiae, especially after posteriorly placed burns, or a narrow drainage angle
Late IOP rise due to loss of effect (not infrequent after longer follow-up)

Post-operative management:

- Check the IOP during the first 1-6 hours. If this is not possible, treat with oral CAIs and α_2 agonists to prevent IOP spikes in susceptible patients.
- Topical corticosteroids or non-steroidal anti-inflammatory agent TID or QID for 4-7 days.

Close monitoring is suggested in the following cases: advanced glaucomatous optic nerve damage with severe field loss, one-eyed patients, high pre-laser IOP, exfoliation syndrome, previous laser trabeculoplasty

Results
The outcomes of a number of randomized prospective clinical trials should be taken into account when considering a patient's suitability for laser trabeculoplasty[78-84].
Large independent clinical trials have shown progressive loss of effect over time[85-87].

Alternative laser systems for laser trabeculoplasty:
Those found effective in reducing IOP in glaucoma include trabeculoplasty with continuous wave lasers of red and infrared wavelengths[88], and, recently, a large spot size, high power, low energy Q-switched, frequency doubled neodymium:YAG (532 nm) system[89].

3.5.3 - LASER IRIDOPLASTY[76]

Indication
- To widen the angle approach by shrinking the peripheral iris using a thermal effect.
- Plateau iris syndrome
- In preparation for ALT when the angle approach is narrow, in order to better visualize the TM
- Angle closure in nanophthalmos ·

Preoperative preparation
As for ALT

Contraindications
severe corneal edema or opacification
flat anterior chamber
synechial angle-closure

Lenses
Laser contact lenses
Abraham lens
Goldmann type lens, aiming through the central part, not the mirrors

Laser parameters
Contraction burns
Spot Size: 300-500 mm
Duration: 0.2-0.5 seconds
Power: 200-400 mW
Location: the aiming beam should be directed at the most peripheral portion of the iris

Goal of treatment is contraction of the peripheral iris with flattening of the peripheral iris curvature.
Ideal number of impacts: 20-50 applications over 360° leaving 2 beam diameters between each spot and avoiding visible radial vessels

Complications:
mild iritis
corneal endothelial burns
transient post-operative IOP elevation
posterior synechiae of the pupil
permanent pupil dilation
Postoperative treatment:
topical steroids for 4-7 days
prevention of IOP spikes (see Ch. 3.6.2)

Post-operative management
Some as under 3.5.2

3.5.4 - CYCLOPHOTOCOAGULATION

Indications
When filtration surgery is likely to fail, has failed, or is not feasible.
As an alternative to drainage devices.

Trans scleral[90]

- Nd:YAG (1064 nm)

Divided into contact and non-contact, as well as continuous wave and pulsed laser systems

Non-contact: the laser energy is transmitted through air from a slit lamp delivery system
Contact: transmission directly from the delivery system to the ocular surface via a fiberoptic hand-held probe placed on the conjunctiva
Pulsed: transmits energy at relatively short, predetermined time intervals
Continuous: allows longer sustained energy delivery with time intervals selected by the surgeon

Technique: Peribulbar or retrobulbar injection of a 50:50 mixture of 2% lidocaine and 0.75% bupivicaine with hyaluronidase
Shields' trans-scleral lens
Distance from limbus 1-3 mm (ciliary body should be localized with transillumination)
Applications: 8-25 over 180°, energy 1.5-10J per pulse

- Diode (810 nm)

Technique: Peribulbar or retrobulbar injection of a 50:50 mixture of 2% lidocaine and 0.75% bupivicaine with hyaluronidase
Distance from limbus 0.5-2.0 mm (ciliary body should be localized with transillumination)
Applications: 10-20 over 180°, energy 5-6J per pulse, total treatment per session up to 270° of circumference (avoid 3 and 9 o'clock positions)

Endoscopic

Endoscopic techniques combined with laser technology allow the photocoagulation of ciliary processes not readily visible via the transpupillary route. The approach can be limbal or via the pars plana, using a fiberoptic probe

- Argon laser
- Diode laser

Transpupillary

This procedure is possible only in cases of aniridia, through a large surgical iridectomy or when broad peripheral anterior synechiae cause anterior displacement of the iris.

- Argon laser
- Diode laser

Complications
Persistent inflammation
Loss of BCVA
Phthisis

Post-operative management
Consider analgesia, topical steroids and topical atropine

GENERAL PRINCIPLES

The different techniques of incisional surgeries have different indications depending on the type of glaucoma. Angle closure glaucoma is usually treated by laser iridotomy or peripheral iridectomy. Different surgical techniques can be used depending on:

1. the target IOP chosen for the individual situation
2. the previous history (surgery, medications)
3. the risk profile (i.e. single eye)
4. the preferences of the surgeon

Congenital glaucoma is suited for primary surgery, usually trabeculotomy or goniotomy, or combinations with filtration surgery including antifibrotic agents.
For repeated surgery, cyclodestructive and tube implants are used
See FC XII

TECHNIQUES

Since glaucoma surgery is practiced in different ways by different ophthalmologists, a detailed description of surgical techniques is not within the scope of this text.

For practical treatment of glaucoma it is permitted to use additional medications if the target IOP is not reached by surgery alone. For the scientific evaluation of a surgical method however, success rate in terms of IOP lowering can only be evaluated in the absence of adjunctive medical treatment. The number of preoperative versus postoperative medications may also depend on the variable compliance of the individual patient before and after surgery. For scientific evaluation of a surgical method, it is useful to count the number of "successes" below a defined cut-off line for IOP as in Fig. 3.3 or calculated according to the CIGTS formula[98]or similar methods.

3.6.1 - PENETRATING GLAUCOMA SURGERY

3.6.1.1 - Trabeculectomy

The current operation of choice in POAG is the trabeculectomy, which produces a 'guarded' fistula between the anterior chamber and the subconjunctival space[92]. The introduction of improved operating microscopes, instruments and suture materials, has led to numerous modifications and refinements of the original operation. Modifications include the size, shape and thickness of the scleral flap, limbal or fornix based conjunctival flaps, fixed, releasable or adjustable sutures and the use of antimetabolites and other antiscarring agents to reduce scarring. In the hand of experts the success rate of filtering surgery (alone, or with adjunctive medical therapy) in a previously unoperated eye is reported up to 90% at 2 years; there are large differences however in the criteria used for the definition of success[100-109]. Long-term IOP control is achieved in many cases, although some patients do require further therapy or repeat surgery. Non penetrating forms of filtration surgery are also practiced although the majority of randomised controlled trials suggest that the pressure lowering is not as great as trabeculectomy.

INDICATIONS

1. In cases where other forms of therapy (namely medicine or laser) have failed.
2. In cases where other forms of therapy are not suitable (eg. where compliance or side-effects are a problem) or appropriate medical treatment is not available.
3. In cases where a target pressure is required that cannot be reached with drops and/or laser.
4. In cases which have such a high IOP at presentation that other forms of treatment are unlikely to be successful[95].

Although medical therapy is still the most frequently used primary treatment in glaucoma, modern glaucoma surgery is generally considered a safe and effective method of achieving good IOP control when ALT is not applicable or successful.
The choice of when to perform glaucoma surgery needs to be made in the light of clinical trials which have monitored the long term outcomes of the three methods of treatment for glaucoma[81,103-105]. In the individual patient, a multitude of factors must be taken into account when deciding treatment including compliance, stage of glaucoma etc. What is suitable for one patient may not be ideal for the next. Nevertheless, surgery is being used more frequently at an earlier stage, rather than as a last resort, if inadequate control is achieved by other forms of therapy or if the patient has a high IOP at presentation. Two studies have indicated that in terms of field survival, primary trabeculectomy may be indicated in certain cases[104,105], although a more recent one has had less conclusive results[91]. The ophthalmologist must assess the risks and benefits of early surgery in each individual case with the knowledge of local outcomes with different therapies[108].

LONG-TERM RISKS OF TRABECULECTOMY

Accelerated progression of senile cataracts is frequently seen after filtration surgery. Patients who have undergone a trabeculectomy should be warned about the possible risks of infection of the drainage bleb which may lead to endophthalmitis and blindness if management is delayed. This event is much more common if blebs are interpalpebral or in the lower fornix and a drainage device should be use if the bleb cannot be positioned under the upper lid. Endophthalmitis is also more common if the bleb is thin and cystic - a situation more commonly found with the use of antimetabolites or full thickness filtration procedures. Patients should be advised of the symptoms of a developing blebitis/endophthalmitis including red eye, tearing, discharge or decreased vision and should be warned to seek the help of an ophthalmologist immediately without delay if any of these symptoms develop in the operated eye.

NOTE

Since glaucoma surgery is practiced in different ways by different ophthalmologists, and almost always not in their office, a detailed description of surgical techniques in not within the scope of this text.

3.6.1.2 - Trabeculotomy

Trabeculotomy is generally used for congenital glaucoma and is less effective in adults.

Arguments *in favor* of non-penetrating glaucoma surgery:
- reduction of postoperative hypotony and consecutive complications (macula edema, choroidal effusion, choroidal hemaorrhage, long-term cataract formation)
- reduction of intraoperative complications (iris prolapse, expulsive hemorrhage)
- Viscocanalostomy may reinstitute physiologic outflow routes through Schlemm's canal and collector channels

Arguments *against* non-penetrating glaucoma surgery:
- Less efficient in IOP reduction (mean IOP 2-4 mmHg higher) than after trabeculectomy
- Difficult technique (learning curve)
- Episcleral/conjunctival fibrosis same as trabeculectomy
- Nd:YAG laser gonio puncture often needed for IOP control

Arguments *in favor* of trabeculectomy
- lower long-term postoperative IOP
- fewer IOP-lowering medications needed postoperatively
- better long-term efficacy

Arguments *against* trabeculectomy
- postoperative increase of lens opacities
- postoperative bleb infection

3.6.2 - NON PENETRATING GLAUCOMA SURGERY

These techniques have recently been advocated as operations for primary open-angle glaucoma. Two different modifications are presently used as "non-penetrating" surgery[106-111].

3.6.2.1 - Deep sclerectomy[111-123]

In this technique, a deep lamella of corneosclera underneath the scleral flap is excised thus removing the outer wall of Schlemm's canal. The outer layer of the inner wall of Schlemm's canal is frequently also removed. Percolation of aqueous occurs through the porosity of the remaining trabecular meshwork, possibly through microperforations. When the scleral flap is repositioned, a "scleral lake" is created. A collagen implant or a hyaluronic acid device is often used to keep this scleral lake patent. Usually a filtration bleb forms; long-term IOP control was reported to be less effective than with trabeculectomy[129].

3.6.2.2 - Viscocanalostomy

In this technique hyaluronic acid is injected into Schlemm's canal. The mechanism claimed to increase the outflow is the widening of Schlemm's canal and of the collector channels as well as diffusion of aqueous from the "scleral lake"[124-130].

3.6.3 - METHODS OF PREVENTING FILTERING BLEB SCARRING

3.6.3.1 - Antimetabolites

(See also Ch. 3.7 and FC XIII)

Antimetabolites such as 5-Fluorouracil (5-FU) and Mitomycin-C (MMC) are now used frequently in patients undergoing glaucoma filtration surgery in order to reduce scarring and improve drainage. The use of these substances is being refined, following the outcome of several studies. Indications and technique needs to be carefully adhered to[131]. Risk factors for scarring include previous ocular surgery, long-term topical medications particularly those that cause a red eye[35,132], young age, black race, uveitis, neovascular glaucoma and others. The risk of corneal epithelial erosions, epitheliopathy, late hypotony, bleb leaks and bleb infections must be considered. New compounds are being investigated to more specifically target the biological processes causing excessive scarring, with the aim of reducing complications[133].

3.6.3.2 - Alternative methods of preventing filtering bleb scarring

Irradiation

Irradiation by various types of radiation was used during the 1970s and has proven to be effective. However, long-term effects on the lens and on the retinal vessels (radiation retinopathy) have to be considered.

Photodynamic therapy

A dye is injected subconjunctivally at the site of operation, resulting in incorporation of the dye into the fibroblasts of the filtering bleb area. A blue light is then irradiated that will selectively destroy the fibroblasts.

Inhibition of growth factors

Recently, attention has been turned to the role of cytokines in the process of wound healing. TGFß2 has been identified as a probable key cytokine in post trabeculectomy wound healing. Human monoclonal anti-TGFß2 antibodies are being tested and pilot studies have shown promising results[133]. Other approaches are also considered such as TGFß2 anti-sense nucleotides, suramine and others.

3.6.4 - COMPLEX CASES

Complicated glaucoma cases such as those that have failed previous surgery, glaucoma secondary to uveitis, rubeosis, retinal surgery, congenital glaucomas, etc. require specialist treatment.

In addition to trabeculectomy, other forms of therapy may be necessary such as glaucoma drainage devices, and ciliary body ablation with the diode laser ("cyclodiode"), free running YAG laser ("cyclo YAG") or cryoprobe ("cyclocryotherapy"). (see Ch. 3.6.4, 3.7.5 and FC XII)

3.6.5 - DRAINAGE DEVICES

The use of drainage devices such as those described by Molteno[134-139], Krupin[140], Baerveldt[141-144], Ahmed[145-148] or Sbocket[149] is generally reserved for patients with risk factors for a poor result with trabeculectomy with antimetabolite.
These factors include previous failed filtering surgery with antimetabolites, excessive conjunctival scarring due to previous surgery,with severe conjunctival or surface disease, active neovascular disease, paediatric aphakia, or where filtration surgery is going to be technically difficult[134-150].

A number of other devices aimed at replacing conventional filtering surgery for POAG are in different stages of development[151-152].

3.7 - ANTIMETABOLITES IN GLAUCOMA FILTERING SURGERY

See also Ch. 3.6.3.1 and FC XIII

Antimetabolites are used to reduce scarring at the site of trabeculectomy[131,153-158]. Healing and scarring are the main determinant of the long term intraocular pressure control after trabeculectomy[169-163].

Aim: - to prevent postoperative conjunctival scarring with resultant failure of filtration
- to reach a low target pressure

Increaded risk for scarring:

- Neovascular glaucoma
- Previous failed glaucoma filtration surgery
- Previous cataract surgery (conjunctival incision)
- Aphakia (intracapsular surgery)
- Recent intraocular surgery (< 3 months)
- Inflammatory eye disease e.g. uveitis, ocular pemphigoid, Stevens-Johnson Syndrome,
- Afro-Caribbean / Hispanic race
- Young age
- Chronic topical medications

<u>Drugs used:</u>

<u>5-Fluorouracil:</u>

Dose: 5 mg. It is available in 25 and 50 mg/ml concentrations. 50 mg/ml now by far the most commonly used. Administered intra- or post-operatively.

Intraoperative use:	Administrated intra operatively on a filter paper or a sponge 25 or 50 mg/ml undiluted solution Time of exposure usually 5 minutes (shorter time has minimal effect with 5-FU) Rinse with approximately 20 ml of balanced salt solution
Post-operative use	Relative contraindication if epithelial problems present 5 mg injections. 0.1ml of 50 mg/ml undiluted solution Small calibre needle (e.g. 30 G needle on insulin syringe) Adjacent to but not into bleb (pH 9) Multiple injections possible - some evidence that less than a total of 3 injections has a minimal impact on scarring

<u>Mitomycin C</u>:

Dose: 0,1-0,5 mg/ml. Available in different preparation; care must be taken in diluting it to the desired concentration. Administered intra- operatively, or postoperatively[165-170].

Intraoperative use:	Concentration: 0.2 - 0.4 mg/ml Administered intraoperatively on a filter paper or a sponge for 2-5 minutes Avoid contact with cut edge of conjunctive flap After application rinse with approximately 20 ml of balanced salt solution

Post-operative use	Concentration: 0.2 mg/ml 0.02 mg injections. Small calibre needle (e.g. 30 G needle on insulin syringe) Adjacent to but not into bleb Multiple injections possible - some evidence that less than a total of 3 injections has a minimal impact

GENERAL PRINCIPLES

The use of cytotoxics increases the requirement for accurate surgery. If aqueous flow is not well controlled persistent hypotony will occur. Strategies to increase control of flow include smaller sclerostomies, larger scleral flaps and releaseable or adjustable sutures.

Recent research has suggested that a large surface area of cytotoxic treatment together with large scleral flaps and fornix based conjunctival flaps leads to diffuse, posteriorly extended non-cystic blebs with a considerable reduction in bleb related complications such as blebitis and endophthalmitis[160-161].
Start with weaker agents (e.g. 5-FU rather than MMC) and lower concentrations (of MMC) until familiar with these agents

CAUTION

Do not allow cytotoxic agents to enter the eye. 5-FU has a pH of 9.0. One drop (0.05ml) of MMC would cause irreversible endothelial damage.

Observe precautions for cytotoxic use and disposal

<u>Complications</u>:
Corneal epitheliopathy (5FU)
Wound Leak
Bleb leak
Hypotony
Blebitis
Endophthalmitis

IMPORTANT: assess each individual case for risk factors, and/or for the need of low target IOP and titrate the substance and dosage used accordingly based on local experience

5-FU and MMC are not officially approved for direct ocular applications. Their use in selected cases as adjunctives in filtration surgery, however, has become standard clinical practice.

References

1) Sommer A, Tielsch JM, Katz J, Quigley HA, Gottsch JD, Javitt J, Singh K. Relationship between intraocular pressure and primary open-angle glaucoma among white and black Americans. The Baltimore Eye Survey. Arch Ophthalmol 1991;109:1090-1095.
2) Tielsch JM, Katz J, Singh K, Quigley HA, Gottsch JD, Javitt J, Sommer A. A population-based evaluation of glaucoma screening. Am J Epidemiol 1991;134:1102-1110.
3) Leske MC, Wu SY, Nemesure B, Hennis A. Incident open-angle glaucoma and blood pressure. Arch Ophthalmol 2002;120:954-959.
4) Butt Z, McKillop G, O'Brien C, Allan P. Measurement of ocular blood flow velocity using colour Doppler imaging in low tension glaucoma. Eye 1995;9:29-33.
5) Bojic L, Skare-Librenjak L. Circulating platelet aggregates in glaucoma. In Ophthalmol 1999;22:151-155.
6) Costa VP, Sergott RC, Smith M, Spaeth GL, Wilson RP, Moster MR, et al. Color Doppler imaging in glaucoma patients with asymmetric optic cups. J Glaucoma 1994;3 Suppl 1:S91-97.
7) Drance SM, Douglas GR, Wijsman K, Schulzer M, Britton RJ. Response of blood flow to warm and cold in normal and low-tension glaucoma patients. Am J Ophthalmol 1988;105:35-39.
8) Flammer J, Guthauser U, Mahler F. Do ocular vasospasms help cause lowtension glaucoma? Doc Ophthalmol Proc Seri 1987;49:397-399.
9) Galassi F, Nuzzaci G, Sodi A, CasiP, Vielmo A. Color Doppler imaging in evaluation of optic nerve blood supply in normal and glaucomatous subjects. Int Ohthalmol 1992;16:273-276.
10) Graham SL, Drance SM, Wijsman K, Mikelberg FS, Douglas GR. Nocturnal hypotension in glaucoma patients. Invest Ophthalmol Vis Sci 1993;34:1286.
11) Graham SL, Drance SM. Nocturnal Hypotension. Role in glaucoma progression. Surv Ophthalmol 1999;43 suppl 1:S10-16.
12) Guthauser U, Flammer J, Mahler F. The relationship between digital and ocular vasospasm. Graefes Arch Clin Exp Ophthalmol 1988;226:224-226.
13) Flammer J, Orgul S, Costa VP, Orzalesi N, Krieglstein GK, Serra LM, Renard JP, Sefansson E. The impact of ocular blood flow in glaucoma. Progress in retinal and eye research. 2002;21(4):359-393.
14) The AGIS Investigators. The advanced glaucoma intervention study (AGIS): 7. The relationship between control of intraocular pressure and visual field deterioration. Am J Ophthalmol 2000;130:429-440.
15) Kass MA, Heuer DK, Higginbotham EJ et al. The Ocular Hypertension Treatment Study: a randomized trial determines that topical ocular hypotensive medication delays or prevents the onset of primary open-angle glaucoma. Arch Ophthalmol 2002;120:701-713.
16) Heijl A, Leske MC, Bengtsson B, et al. Reduction of intraocular pressure and glaucoma progression: results from the Early Manifest Glaucoma Trial. Arch Ophthalmol 2002; 120: 1268-1279.
17) Leske CM, Heijl A, Hussein M, Bengtsson B, Hyman L, Komaroff E for the Early Manifest Glaucoma Trial Group. Factors for glaucoma progression and the effect of treatmen. The Early Manifest Glaucoma Trial. Arch Ophthalmol 2003;1210:48-569.
18) Wilensky JT, Gieser DK, Dietsche ML, Mori MT, Zeimer R. Individual variability in the diurnal intraocular pressure curve. Ophthalmol 1993;100:940-944.
19) Zeimer RC, Wilensky JT, Gieser DK, Viana MA. Association between intraocular pressure peaks and progression of visual field loss. Ophthalmol 1991;98:64-69.
20) Niesel P, Flammer J. Correlations between intraocular pressure, visual field and visual acuity, based on 11 years of observations of treated chronic glaucomas. Int Ophthal 1980;3:31-35.
21) Flammer J, Eppler E, Niesel P. Quantitative perimetry in glaucoma patient without local visual field defects. Graefe's Arch Clin Exp Ophthalmol 1982;219:92-94.
22) Asrani A et al. Large diurnal fluctuations in intraocular pressure as an independent risk factor in patients with glaucoma. Journal of Glaucoma 2000;9:134-142.
23) Goldberg I. Compliance. In: Ritch R, Shields M B, Krupin T (eds.). The glaucomas. Mosby, St. Louis 1996;1375-1384.
24) Janz NK, Wren PA, Lichter PR, Musch DC, Gillespie BW, Guire KE, The CIGTS Group. Quality of life in diagnosed glaucoma patients. The Collaborative Initial Glaucoma Treatment Study. Ophthalmology 2001;108:887-898.

25) Janz NK, Wren PA, Lichter PR, Musch DC, Gillespie BW, Guire KE, Mills RP, CIGTS Study Group. The Collaborative Initial Glaucoma Treatment Study (CIGTS): Interim Quality of Life Findings Following Initial Medical or Surgical Treatment of Glaucoma. Ophthalmology 2001;108:1954-65.
26) Bigger JF. A comparison of patient compliance in treated vs. untreated ocular hypertension. Trans Am Acad Ophthalmol Otolaryngol. 1976;81:277-285.
27) Cramer JA, Mattson RH, Prevey ML, Scheyer RD, Ouellette VL. How often is medication taken as prescribed? A novel assessment technique. JAMA 1989 Jun 9;261(22):3273-3277.
28) Patel SC, Spaeth GL. Compliance in patients prescribed eyedrops for glaucoma. Ophthalmic Surg 1995;26(3):233-236.
29) Greenberg RN. Overview of patient compliance with medication dosing: a literature review. Clin Ther. 1984;6:592-599.
30) Schuman JS. Antiglaucoma medications: a review of safety and tolerability issues related to their use. Clin Ther 2000;22(2):167-208.
31) Odberg T, Jakobsen JE, Hultgren SJ, Halseide R. The impact of glaucoma on the quality of life of patients in Norway. II. Patient response correlated to objective data. Acta Ophthalmol Scand 2001;79(2):121-124. Comments: Acta Ophthalmol Scand. 2001;79(2):107.
32) Odberg T, Jakobsen JE, Hultgren SJ, Halseide R. The impact of glaucoma on the quality of life of patients in Norway. I. Results from a self-administered questionnaire. Acta ophthalmol Scand 2001;79:116-120.
33) Baudouin C, Nordmann JP, Denis P, Creuzot-Garcher C, Allaire C, Trinquand C. Efficacy of indomethacin 0.1% and fluorometholone 0.1% on conjunctival inflammation following chronic application of antiglaucomatous drugs. Graefes Arch Clin Exp Ophthalmol 2002;240(11):929-935.
34) Pisella PJ, Pouliquen P, Baudouin C. Prevalence of ocular symptoms and signs with preserved and preser - vative free glaucoma medication. Br J Ophthalmol 2002; 86(4):418-423.
35) Baudouin C, Pisella PJ, Fillacier K, Goldschild M, Becquet F, De Saint Jean M, Bechetoille A. Ocular surface inflammatory changes induced by topical antiglaucoma drugs: human and animal studies. Ophthalmology 1999; 106(3):556-563.
36) Goldberg I. Should β blockers be abandoned as initial monotherapy in chronic open-angle glaucoma? The controversy. Br J Ophthalmol 2002;86:691-695.
37) Anton A. Should β blockers be abandoned as initial monotherapy in chronic open-angle glaucoma? View 1. Br J Ophthalmol 2002;86:692-693.
38) Skuta GL. Should β blockers be abandoned as initial monotherapy in chronic open-angle glaucoma? View 2. Br J Ophthalmol 2002;86:693-694.
39) Stamper, RL. Primary drug treatment for glaucoma: Beta-blockers versus other medications for glaucoma. I. Individualize Initial Therapy. Surv Ophthalmol 2002;63-73.
40) Wigginton SA, Higginbotham EJ. Primary drug treatment for glaucoma: Beta-blockers versus other medications for glaucoma. II. Choosing beta-blockers for initial medical therapy for glaucoma. Surv Ophthalmol 2002;63-73.
41) Mittag TW. Adrenergic and dopaminergic drugs in glaucoma. In: Ritch R, Shields MB, Krupin T (eds). The Glaucomas. St. Louis, Mosby, 1989;1409-1424.
42) Gieser SC, Juzych M, Robin AL, Schwartz GF. Clinical pharmacology of adrenergic drugs. In: Ritch R, Shields MB, Krupin T (eds). The Glaucomas. St. Louis, Mosby, 1989;1425-1448.
43) Radius RL. Use of betaxolol in the reduction of elevated intraocular pressure. Arch Ophthalmol 1983;101:898.
44) Nardin GF, Zimmerman TJ. Ocular Cholinergic agents. In: Ritch R, Shields MB, Krupin T (eds). The Glaucomas. St. Louis, Mosby, 1996;66:1399-1409.
45) Drance SM, Nash PA. The dose response of human intraocular pressure to pilocarpine. Can J Ophthalmol 1971;6:9.
46) Lippa EA. Carbonic anhydrase inhibitors. In: Ritch R, Shields MB, Krupin T (eds). The Glaucomas. St. Louis, Mosby, 1996;70:1463-1482.
47) Camras CB. Prostaglandins. In: Ritch R, Shields MB, Krupin T (eds). The Glaucomas. St. Louis, Mosby, 1989;1449-1461.
48) Alm A, Stjernschantz J. Effects on intraocular pressure and side effects of 0.005% latanoprost applied once daily, evening or morning. A comparison with timolol. Scandinavan Latanoprost Study Group. Ophthalmology 1996;103:126-137.

49) Waewar RE, Bullock JD, Ballal D. cystoid macular edema and anterior uveitis associated with latanoprost use. Ophthalmology 1998;105:263-368.
50) Katz LJ. Brimonidine tartrate 0.2% twice daily vs timolol 0.5% twice daily: 1- year results in glaucoma patients. Brimonidine Study Group. Am J Ophthalmol 1999;127:20-26.
51) Gandolfi SA, Cimino L. Effect of bimatoprost on patients with primary open-angle glaucoma or ocular hypertension who are nonresponders to latanoprost. Ophthalmology 2003;110(3):609-614.
52) Hayreh SS, Podhajsky P and Zimmerman MB. Beta-blocker eyedrops and nocturnal arterial hypotension. Am J Ophthalmol 1999;128:301-309.
53) Higginbotham BJ, Schuman JS, Goldberg I, et al. Bimatropost Study Group 1 and 2. One-year randomized study comparing Bimatoprost and Timolol in Glaucoma and ocular hypertension. Arch Ophthalmol 2002;120:1286-1289.
54) Alm A, Camras CB and Watson PG. Phase III latanoprost studies in Scandinavia, the United Kingdom and he United States. Surv Ophthalmol 1997;41 Suppl 2:105-110.
55) Netland PA, Landry T, Sullivan EK, Andrew R, Silver L, Weiner A, Mallick S, Dickerson J, Bergamini MV, Robertson SM, Davis AA. Travoprost compared with latanoprost and timolol in patients with open-angle glaucoma or ocular hypertension. Am J Ophthalmol. 2001;132(4):472-484.
56) Sherwood M, Brandt J. Six-month comparison of bimatoprost once-daily and twice-daily with timolol twice-daily in patients with elevated intraocular pressure. Surv Ophthalmol. 2001;45 Suppl 4:S361-368.
57) Brubaker RF, Schoff EO, Nau CB et al. Effects of AGN 192024, a new ocular hypotensive agent, on aqueous dynamics. Am J Ophthalmol 2001;11:19-24.
58) Noecker RS, Dirks MS, Choplin NT, Bernstein P, Batoosingh AL and Whitcup SM for the Bimatoprost/Latanoprost Study Group. A Six-Months Randomized Clinical Trial Comparing the IOP-Lowering Efficacy of Bimatoprost and Latanoprost in Patients With Ocular Hypertension or Glaucoma. Am J Ophthalmol 2003.
59) K. Parrish R, Palmberg P, Sheu WP for the XLT Study Group. A Comparison of Latanoprost, Bimatoprost and Travoprost in Patients with elevated intraocular pressure: A 12-week, randomized, masked-evaluator, Multicenter Study. Am J Ophthalmol, 2003.
60) Sherwood M, Brandt J. Six-month comparison of bimatoprost once-daily and twice-daily with timolol twice-daily in patients with elevated intraocular pressure. Surv Ophthalmol. 2001;45 Suppl 4:S361-368.
61) Azuma I, Masuda K, Kitazawa Y, Yamamura H. Double-masked comparative study of UF-021 and timolol ophthalmic solutions in patients with primary open-angle glaucoma or ocular hypertension. Jpn J Ophthalmol 1993;37:514-525.
62) Wistrand PJ, Stjernschantz J, Olsson K. The incidence and time-course of latanoprost-induced iridial pigmentation as a function of eye color. Surv Ophthalmol 1997;41(Suppl 2):S129-138.
63) Yamamoto T, Kitazawa Y. Iris-color change developed after topical isopropyl unoprostone treatment. J Glaucoma 1997;6:430-432.
64) Brown SM. Increased iris pigment in a child due to latanoprost. Arch Ophthalmol 1998;116:1683-1684.
65) Wand M. Latanoprost and hyperpigmentation of eyelashes. Arch Ophthalmol 1997;115:1206-1208.
66) Sudesh S, Cohen EJ, Rapuano CJ, Wilson RP. Corneal toxicity associated with latanoprost. Arch Ophthalmol 1999;117:539-540.
67) Wand M, Gilbert CM, Liesegang TJ. Latanoprost and herpes simplex keratitis. Am J Ophthalmol 1999;127:602-604.
68) Warwar RE, Bullock JD. Latanoprost-induced uveitis. Surv Ophthalmol 1999;43:466-468.
69) Miyake K, Ota I, Maekubo K, et al. Latanoprost accelerates disruption of the blood-aqueous barrier and the incidence of angiographic cystoid macular edema in early postoperative pseudophakias. Arch Ophthalmol 1999;117:34-40.
70) Moroi SE, Gottfredsdottir MS, Schteingart MT, et al. Cystoid macular edema associated with latanoprost therapy in a case series of patients with glaucoma and ocular hypertension. Ophthalmology 1999;106:1024-1029.
71) Waldock A, Snape J, Graham CM. Effects of glaucoma medications on the cardiorespiratory and intraocular pressure status of newly diagnosed glaucoma patients. Br J Ophthalmol 2000;84:710-713.
72) Diestelhorst M, Almegard B. Comparison of two fixed combinations of latanoprost and timolol in open-angle glaucoma. Graefes Arch Clin Exp Ophthalmol 1998;236(8):577-581.
73) Sponsel WE, Paris G, Trigo Y, Pena M. Comparative effects of latanoprost (Xalaton™) and unoprostone

(Rescula™) in patients with glaucoma and with suspected glaucoma. Am J Ophthalmol 2002;134:552-559.
74) Choudhri S, Wand M, Shields MB. Comparison of dorzolamide-timolol fixed combination therapy to concomitant administration of a topical beta-blocker and dorzolamide. Am J Ophthalmol. 2000;130:832.
75) Hoskins H D Jr, Kass M. Becker-Shaffer' Diagnosis and therapy of the glaucomas. St. Louis, C.V. Mosby 1989;412-419.
76) Ritch R, Liebmann JM. Laser iridotomy and peripheral iridoplasty. In: Ritch R, Shields M B, Krupin T (eds.). The glaucomas. St. Louis, Mosby 1996;1594-1577.
77) Weinreb RN, Tsai CS. Laser trabeculoplasty. In: Ritch R, Shields MB, Krupin T (eds.) The Glaucomas. St. Louis, Mosby 1996;1575-1590.
78) Migdal C, Gregory W, Hitchings RA. Long-term functional outcome after early surgery compared with laser and medicine in open-angle glaucoma. Ophthalmology 1994;101:1651-1657.
79) The Glaucoma Laser Trial Research Group. The Glaucoma Laser Trial (GLT). 2. Results of argon laser trabe culoplasty versus topical medicines. Ophthalmology 1990;97:1403-1413.
80) The Glaucoma Laser Trial Research Group. The Glaucoma Laser Trial[87] (GLT). 6. Treatment group differences in visual field changes. Am J Ophthalmol 1995;120:10-22.
81) The Glaucoma Laser Trial Research Group. The Glaucoma Laser Trial Follow-up Study. (GLT). 7. Results. Am J Ophthalmol 1995;120:718-731.
82) The AGIS Investigators. The Advanced Glaucoma Intervention Study (AGIS: 4). Comparison of treatment outcomes within race. Seven-year results. Ophthalmology 1998;105:1146-1164.
83) The AGIS Investigators. The Advanced Glaucoma Intervention Study (AGIS): 6. Effect of cataract on visual field and visual acuity. Arch Ophthalmol 2000;118:1639-1652.
84) The AGIS Investigators. The Advanced Glaucoma Intervention Study (AGIS)[91]: 9. Comparison of glaucoma outcomes in black and white patients within treatment groups. Am J Ophthalmol 2001;132:311-320.
85) Spaeth GL, Baez K. Argon laser trabeculoplasty control one third of cases of progressive, uncontrolled, open-angle glaucoma for 5 years. Arch Ophthalmol 1992;110:491.
86) The glaucoma Laser trial research group: the glaucoma trail. 1. Acute effects of argon laser trabeculoplasty on intraocular pressure. Arch Ophthalmol 1989;107:1135.
87) Eendebak GR, Boen-Tan TN, Bezemer PD. Long-term follow-up of laser trabeculoplasty. Doc Ophthalmol 1990;75:203.
88) Moriarty AP, McHugh JDA, Fytche TJ, Marshall J, Hamilton AMP. Long-term follow-up of diode laser trabeculoplasty for primary open-angle glaucoma and ocular hypertension. Ophthalmology 1993;100:1614-1618.
89) Latina MA, Sibayan SA, Shin DH, Noecker RJ, Marcellino G. Q-switched 532-nm Nd:YAG laser trabeculoplasty (Selective Laser Trabeculoplasty). A multicenter pilot clinical study. Ophthalmology 1998;105:2082-2090.
90) Bloom PA, Tsai JC, Sharma K, Miller M H, Rice NASC, Hitchings RA, Khaw PT. Trans-scleral diode laser cyclophotocoagulation in the treatment of advanced refractory glaucoma. Ophthalmology 1997;104:1508-1520.
91) Lichter PR, Musch DC, Gillespie BW, Guire KE, Janz NK, Wren PA, Mills RP, CIGTS Study Group. Interim Clinical Outcomes in the Collaborative Initial Glaucoma Treatment Study (CIGTS) Comparing Initial Treatment Randomized to Medications or Surgery. Ophthalmology 2001;108:1943-1953.
92) Cairns JE. Trabeculectomy. Preliminary report of a new method. Am J Ophthalmol 1968;5:673-679.
93) Nouri-Mahdavi K, Brigatti L, Weitzman M, Caprioli J. Outcomes of trabeclectomy for primary open-angle glaucoma. Ophthalmology l995;102:1760-1769.
94) Mills KB. Trabeculectomy. A retrospective long-term follow-up of 444 case. Br J Ophthalmol 1981;65:790-795.
95) Watson PG, Grierson I. The place of trabeculectomy in the treatment of glaucoma. Ophthalmol 1981;88:175-196.
96) Wilson P. Trabeculectomy: Long-term follow-up. Br J Ophthalmol 1977;61:117-119.
97) Inaba Z. Long-term results of trabeculectomy in the Japanese: An analysis by life-table method. Jpn J Ophthalmol 1982;26:361-373.
98) Molteno ACB, Bosma NJ, Kittelson JM. Otago glaucoma surgery outcome study. Long-term results of trabeculectomy 1976 to 1995. Ophthalmology 1999;106:1742-1750.
99) Diestelhorst M, Khalili MA, Krieglstein GK. Trabeculectomy: a retrospective follow-up of 700 eyes. Int Ophthalmol 1999;22:211-220.
100) Robinson DIM, Lertsumitkul S, Billson FA, Robinson LP. Long-term intraocular pressure control by trabeculectomy; a ten-year life table. Aust N Z J Ophthalmol 1993;21:79-85.
101) D'Ermo F, Bonomi L, Doro D. A critical analysis of the long-term results of trabeculectomy. Am J Ophthalmol

1979;88:829-835.
102) Akafo SK, Goulstine DB, Rosenthal AR. Long-term post trabeculectomy intraocular pressures. Acta Ophthalmol 1992;70:312-316.
103) Lamping KA, Bellows AR, Hutchinson BT, Afran SI. Long-term evaluation of initial filtration surgery. Ophthalmology 1986;93:91-101.
104) Jay JL, Murray SB. Early trabeculectomy versus conventional management in primary open-angle glaucoma. Brit J Ophthalmol 1988;72:881-889.
105) Migdal C, Gregory W, Hitchings RA. Long-term functional outcome after early surgery compared with laser and medicine in open-angle glaucoma. Ophthalmology 1994;101:1651-1657.
106) Tan JCH, Hitchings RA. Non-penetrating glaucoma surgery: the state of the play. Br J Ophthalmol 2001:85:234-237.
107) Netland PA, Ophthalmic Technology Assessment. Non-penetrating glaucoma surgery. Ophthalmology 2001;108:416-421.
108) Bhandari A, Crabb DP, Poinoosawmy D, Fitzke FW, Hitchings RA, Noureddin BN. Effect of surgery on visual field progression in normal-tension glaucoma. Ophthalmology 1997;104:1131-1137.
109) Mermoud A, Schnyder CC. Non-penetrating filtering surgery in glaucoma. Curr Opin Ophthalmol 2002;11:151-157.
110) Johnson DH, Johso MJ. How does non-penetrating glaucoma surgery work? Aqueous outflow resistance and glaucoma surgery. J Glaucoma 2001;10:55-67.
111) Krieglstein GK. How new is new, and is it better? J Glaucoma 1999;8:279-280.
112) El Sayyad F, Helal M, El-Kholfy H, Khalil M, El-Maghraby A. Non-penetrating deep sclerectomy versus trabeculectomy in bilateral primary open-angle glaucoma. Ophthalmology 2000;107:1671-1674.
113) Di Staso S, Taverniti L, Genitti G, Marangolo L, Aiello A, Giuffre L, Balestrazzi E. Combined phacoemulsification and deep sclerectomy vs phacoemulsification and trabeculectomy. Acta Ophthalmol Scand Suppl 2000;232:59-60.
114) Mermoud A, Schnyder CC, Sickenberg M, Chiou AG, Hediguer SE. Comparison of deep sclerectomy with collagen implant and trebeculectomy in open-angle glaucoma. J Cataract Refract Surg 1999;25(3):323-331.
115) Sanchez E, Schnyder CC, Sickenberg M, Chiou AGY, Hediguer SEA, Mermoud A. Deep sclerectomy: results with and without implant. Int Ophthalmol 1997;20:157-162.
116) Demailly P, Lavat P, Kretz G, Jeanteur-Lunel MN. Non-penetrating deep sclerectomy (NPDS) with or without collagen device (CD) in primary open-angle glaucoma: middle-term retrospective study. Int Ophthalmol 1997;20:131-140.
117) Karlen ME, Sanchez E, Schnyder CC, Sickenberg M, Mermoud A. Deep sclerectomy with collagen implant: medium term results. Br J Ophthalmol 1999;83:6-11.
118) Dahan E, Drusedau MUH. Non-penetrating filtration surgery for glaucoma: Control by surgery only. J Cataract Refract Surg 2000;26:695-701.
119) Sourdille PH, Santiago PY, Villain F, Yamamichi M, Tahi H, Parel JM, Decournau Y. Reticulated hyaluronic acid implant in nonperforating trabecular surgery. J Cataract Refract Surg 1999;25:332-339.
120) Chiselita D. Non-penetrating deep sclerectomy versus trabeculectomy in primary open-angle glaucoma surgery. Eye 2000;15:197-201.
121) Zimmerman TJ, Kooner KS, Ford VJ, Olander KW. Mandlekorn RM. Rawlings EF, Leader BJ, Koskan AJ. Trabeculectomy vs. non-penetrating trabeculectomy: A Retrospective study of two procedures in phakic patients with glaucoma. Ophthalmic Surg 1984;15:44-50.
122) Gianoli F, Schnyder CC, Bovey E, Mermoud A. Combined surgery for cataract and glaucoma: Phacoemulsification and deep sclerectomy compared with phacoemulsification and trabeculectomy. J Cataract Refrct Surg 1999;25:340-346.
123) Chiou AGY, Mermoud A, Jewelewicz DA. Post-operative inflammation following deep sclerectomy with collagen implant versus standard trabeculectomy. Graefe's Arch Clin Exp Ophthalmol 1998;236:593-596.
124) Carassa RG, Bettin P, Brancato R. Viscocanalostomy: A pilot study. Acta Ophthalmol Scand Suppl 1998;227:51-52.
125) Carassa RG, Bettin P, Fiori M, Brancato R. Viscocanalostomy: A pilot study. Eur J ophthalmol 1998;8:57-61.
126) Welsh NH, DeLange J, Wasserman P, Ziemba SL. The deroofing of Schelmm's canal in patients with open-angle glaucoma through placement of a collagen drainage device. Ophthalmic Surg Lasers 1998;29:216-226.
127) Jonescu-Cuypers C, Jacobi PH, Konen W, Krieglstein GK. Primary viscocanalostomy versus trabeculectomy

in white patients with open-angle glaucoma. Ophthalmology 2001;108:254-258.
128) Stegmann R, Pienaar A, Miller D. Viscocanalostomy for open-angle glaucoma in black African patients. J Cataract Refract Surg 1999;25:316-322.
129) Mermoud A. Sinustomy and deep sclerectomy. Eye 2000;14:531-535.
130) Van Buskirk EM. The sartorial spector of viscocanalostomy. J Glaucoma 2001;10:1-3.
131) Khaw PT, Migdal CS. Current techniques in wound healing modulation in glaucoma surgery. Current Opin. Ophthalmology 1996;7:24-33.
132) Lavin MJ, Wormald RPL, Migdal C, Hitchings RA. The influence of prior therapy on the success of trabeculectomy. Arch. Ophthalmol 1990;108:1543-1548.
133) Siriwardena D, Khaw PT, King AJ, Donaldson ML, Overton BM, Migdal G, Cordeiro MF. Human Antitrasforming Growth Factor β2 Monoclonal Antibody. A new modulator of wound healing in Trabeculectomy. A randomized placebo controlled clinical study. Ophthalmology 2002;109:427-431.
134) Mills RP, Reynolds A, Edmond MJ, Barlow WE, Leen MM. Long-term survival of Molteno glaucoma drainage devices. Ophthalmology 1996;103:299-305.
135) Molteno ACB, Sayawat N, Herbison P. Otago glaucoma surgery outcome study. Long-term results of uveitis with secondary glaucoma drained by Molteno implants. Ophthalmology 2001;108:605-613.
136) Airaksinen PJ, Aisala P, Tuulonen A. Molteno implant surgery in uncontrolled glaucoma. Acta Ophthalmol 1990;68:690-694.
137) Freedman J, Rubin B. Molteno implants as a treatment for refractory glaucoma in black patients. Arch Ophthalmol 1991;109:1417-1420.
138) Price FW Jr, Wellemeyer M. Long-term results of Molteno implants. Ophthalmic Sur 1995;26:130-135.
139) Perkins TW, Gangnon R, Ladd W, Kaufman PL, Libby CM. Molteno implant with mitomycin C: Intermediate-term results. J Glaucoma 1998;7:86-92.
140) Fellenbaum PS, Almeida AR, Minckler DS, Sidoti PA, Baerveldt G, Hever DK. Krupin disc implants for complicated glaucomas. Ophthalmology 1994;101:1178-1182.
141) Britt MT, LaBree LD, Lloyd MA, Minckler DS, Heuer DK, Baerveldt G, Varma R. Randomized clinical trial of the 350-mm2 versus the 500-mm2 Baerveldt implant: longer term results: is bigger better? Ophthalmology 1999;106(12):212-218.
142) Krishna R, Godfrey DG, Budenz DL, et al. Intermediate-term outcomes of 350 mm2 Baerveldt Glaucoma Implants. Ophthalmology 2001;108:621-626.
143) Siegner SW, Netland PA, Urban RC Jr, et al. Clinical experience with the Baerveldt glaucoma drainage implant. Ophthalmology 1995;102:1298-1307.
144) Roy S, Ravinet E, Mermoud A. Baerveldt implant in refractory glaucoma: long-term results and factors influencing outcome. Int Ophthalmol 2001;24:93-100.
145) Coleman AL, Hill R, Wilson MR et al. Initial clinical experience with the Ahmed glaucoma valve implant. Am. J. Ophthalmol 1995;120:23-31.
146) Huang MC, Netland PA, Coleman AL, et al. Intermediate-term clinical experience with the Ahmed glaucoma Valve implant. Am J Ophthalmol 1999;127:27-33.
147) Topouzis F, Coleman AL, Choplin N, et al. Follow-up of the original cohort with the Ahmed glaucoma valve implant. Am J Ophthalmol 1999;128:198-204.
148) Wilson MR, Mendis U, Smith SD, Paliwal A. Ahmed glaucoma valve implant vs trabeculectomy in the surgical treatment of glaucoma: a randomized clinical trial. Am J Ophthalmol 2000;130:267-273.
149) Omi CA, De Almeida GV, Cohen R, et al. Modified Schocket implant for refractory glaucoma. Experience of 55 cases. Ophthalmology 1991;98:211-214.
150) Kwon YH, Taylor JM, Hong S, Honkanen RA, et al. Long-term results of eyes with penetrating keratoplasty and glaucoma drainage tube implant. Ophthalmology 2001;108:272-278.
151) Gandolfi S, Traverso CE, Bron A, Sellem E, Kaplan-Messas A, Belkin M. Short-term results of a miniature draining implant for glaucoma in combined surgery with phacoemulsification. Acta Ophthalmol Scand Suppl 2002; 236:66.
152) Spiegel D, Kobvch K. Trabecular Meshwork bypass tube shunt: initial case series Br J Ophthalmol 2002; 86:1228-1231.
153) Weinreb RN. Adjusting the dose of 5-fluorouracil after filtration surgery to minimize side effects. Ophthalmology 1987;94:564-570.
154) Feldman RM, Dietze PJ, Gross RL, Osman O. Intraoperative 5-Fluorouracil administration in trabeculec-

tomy. J. Glaucoma 1994;3:302-307.
155) Hurvitz LM. 5FU supplemented phacoemulsification, posterior chamber lens implantation and trabeculectomy. Ophthalmic Surg 1993;24:674-680.
156) Kitazawa Y, Kawase K, Matsushita H, Minobe M. Trabeculectomy with mitomycin. A comparative study with fluorouracil. Arch Ophthalmol 1991;109:1693-1698.
157) Heuer DK, Parrish RK 2d, Gressel MG, Hodapp E, Palmberg PF, Anderson DR. 5-fluorouracil and glaucoma filtering surgery. II. A pilot study. Ophthalmology 1984;91:384-394.
158) Shin DH, Kim YY, Sheth N, Ren J, Shah M, Kim C, Yang KJ. The role of adjunctive mitomicin C in secondary glaucoma triple procedure as compared to primary glaucoma triple procedure. Ophthalmology 1998;105:740-745.
159) Wells A, Cordeiro M, Bunce CV, and Khaw PT. Cystic bleb related complications in limbus versus fornix based flaps in paediatric and young adult trabeculectomy with high dose mitomycin C. Invest Ophthalmol Vis Sci 2001;42(4):S544
160) Khaw PT, Wilkins M. Antifibrotic agents in glaucoma surgery. In: Yanof M, Dueker JS (eds.). Ophthalmology. London, Mosby 1998;12:31.1-31.8.
161) Khaw PT, Wells AP, Lim KS. Surgery for glaucoma in the 21st century. Br J Ophthalmol 2002;86(7):710-711.
162) Iester M, Ravinet E, Mermoud A. Postoperative subcongiuntival Mitomycin-C injection after non-penetrating glaucoma surgery. J Ocular Pharmacol Ther 2002;18:307-312.
163) Mietz A, Jacobi PC, Krieglstein GK. Postoperative application of mitomycin for trabeculectomies. Arch Ophthalmol 2000;18:1341-1348.
164) Cordeiro MF. Beyond Mitomicin: TGF β and wound healing - progress in retina and eye research 2002;21:75-89.

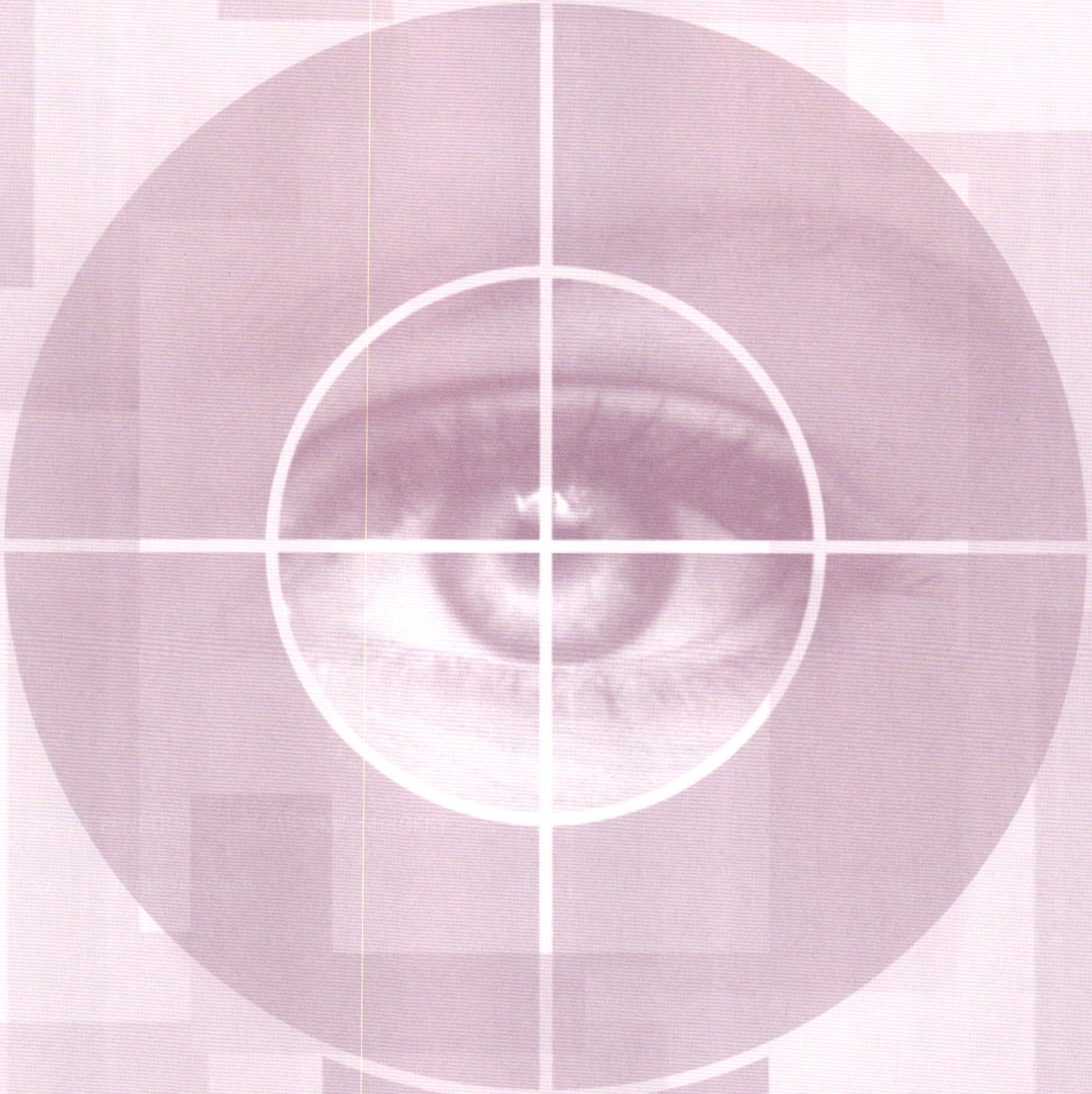

CHAPTER 4

TREATMENT GUIDELINES

4.1 - PRIMARY CONGENITAL FORMS

Medical treatment is usually not effective nor practicable in long term. Medications, including oral CAIs can be considered in preparation for surgery, and in case of failed surgery while awaiting for further options.

4.1.1 - PRIMARY CONGENITAL GLAUCOMA

* Primary surgery: early goniotomy or trabeculotomy or filtration surgery may be indicated as IOP rise results from trabecular maldevelopment

4.1.2 - PRIMARY INFANTILE GLAUCOMA

* Primary surgery: early goniotomy or trabeculotomy or filtration surgery

4.1.3 - GLAUCOMA ASSOCIATED WITH CONGENITAL ANOMALIES

* Treatment to be adapted to the primary anomaly, the mechanism of IOP elevation and the quality of life of the patient

4.2 - PRIMARY OPEN-ANGLE GLAUCOMAS

4.2.1 - PRIMARY JUVENILE GLAUCOMA

a) Medical therapy: any effective and well tolerated topical regimen.
Pilocarpine causes fluctuating myopic shift, visual symptoms and headache particularly in the young and should be avoided.
b) Surgery: early surgery recommended
filtering procedure or trabeculotomy; consider antimetabolites
c) Laser trabeculoplasty: not recommended due to poor and short-lived IOP lowering effect

4.2.2 - PRIMARY JUVENILE GLAUCOMA SUSPECT

* The indication for therapy is relative
* No well-documented scientific clinical trials with well-defined guidelines for treatment

The risk of developing glaucoma increases with the number and strength of risk factors.

The likelihood that these risk factors will contribute to the development of glaucomatous optic nerve damage should be carefully weighed against the risks of treatment (see Ch. 2.2).

The potential benefit of treatment should outweigh the negative side effects of therapy on the patient's vision, general health and quality of life since life expectancy is long.
a) Medical therapy: if indicated, same as for primary juvenile glaucoma
b) Surgery: not indicated
c) Laser trabeculoplasty not recommended due to poor and short-lived IOP lowering effect
d) Follow-up at intervals of 6-12 months with examination of:
- Optic disc
- Visual field
- IOP
- Optic Disc and/or Retinal Nerve Fibre Layer photographs or imaging initially and every 2-3 years

If negative, F/U interval can be increased to 12-18 months

4.2.3 - PRIMARY OPEN-ANGLE GLAUCOMA (POAG/HPG)

Refer also to Introduction II and Ch. 3.1

A target pressure is to be identified for each case (See also Ch. 3.1.1, 3.2 and FC)
It is essential to involve the patient as an informed partner in decisions regarding management of their status.
a) Medical treatment (see Flow Charts)
1. Mono therapy
2. Combination therapy when needed in selected patients
b) Laser trabeculoplasty (LTP)
c) Filtration Surgery with / without antimetabolites
Adjunctive medical therapy when needed
d) Insertion of aqueous drainage tubes / setons
e) Cyclodestructive procedures

Choice of primary therapeutic modality needs to be made on an individual patient basis.

4.2.4 - PRIMARY OPEN-ANGLE GLAUCOMA SUSPECT (POAG/HPG SUSPECT)

Risks and benefits of treatment need to be weighed against the risk of the development of glaucomatous disc damage. The risk of developing glaucoma increases with the number and strength of risk factors.
It is essential to involve the patient as a informed partner in decisions regarding management of their status.

Management: The indication for any form of therapy is relative

a) Medical therapy: any topical agent alone or in combination as long as well tolerated and effective
Avoid adjunctive medical treatment unless strictly needed
b) Laser trabeculoplasty: not usually indicated
c) Filtering operation: not indicated
d) Follow-up at intervals of 6 months initially, to be increased if all parameters remain normal with examination of:

- Optic disc
- Visual field
- IOP
- ONH and RNFL photographs initially and every 2-3 years

4.2.5 - NORMAL-PRESSURE GLAUCOMA (POAG/NPG)

(See Introduction II and Ch. 3.1)
There are few prospective clinical trials indicating clearly the advantages of treatment.
Target pressure: in most cases a peak IOP = 8 mm - 15 mm Hg on diurnal curve

or

a 30% IOP reduction from baseline (see Ch. 3.2)

a) Medical therapy: Any drug effective and tolerated, sufficient to reach the target IOP. Avoid medications with potential vasoconstrictive effects or with systemic hypotensive effects i.e. non selective betablockers. Oral calcium channel blockers are being investigated in selected patients.
b Laser trabeculoplasty
c) Surgery: in cases of progressive glaucomatous damage, in spite of maximal medical therapy or laser trabeculoplasty, or failure to reach target pressure. Intensive postoperative care with bleb manipulation may be needed to maintain low IOPs.

Follow-up at intervals of 3 -12 months, with examination of:

- Optic disc
- Visual field
- IOP
- ONH and RNFL photographs initially and every 2-3 years

4.2.6 - NORMAL-PRESSURE GLAUCOMA SUSPECT (POAG/NPG SUSPECT)

Observe theses patients carefully.
Treatment is not indicated unless there is suggestion of disease progression. If disease progression is due to glaucoma, manage as under 4.2.5
a) Medical therapy indicated only when visual field / optic nerve head are worsening: use any drug effective and tolerated sufficient to reach the target IOP. Avoid medications with potential vasoconstrictive effects or with systemic hypotensive effects
b) Laser Trabeculoplasty: not indicated.
c) Filtering surgery: not indicated.

Follow-up at intervals of 3 -12 months, with examination of:

- Optic disc
- Visual field
- IOP
- ONH and RNFL photographs initially and every 2-3 years

4.2.7 - OCULAR HYPERTENSION (OH)

Although in the past it has been used as a diagnosis, Ocular Hypertension should be used to indicate that the IOP is *consistently* outside 2 standard deviations above the mean. Consider corneal thickness (see Introduction II and Ch. 1.1; FC II and IV).
A modest increase in IOP is not sufficient reason for treatment, but consider it in patients with repeated IOPs in the high twenties, even without risk factors. For treatment modality see Ch. 4.2.3-a. (See also Ch. 2.2.3. and flow-charts)

-If left untreated[Ch. Introduction II]

* up to 9.5% develop glaucoma over 5 year of follow-up
* the risk of developing glaucoma increases with increasing IOP
* prophylactic IOP-lowering therapy to be discussed with individual patients considering the presence of risk factors

Follow-up at intervals of 12 months initially, to be increased if all parameters remain negative, with exami nation of:

- Optic disc
- Visual field
- IOP
- ONH and RNFL photographs initially and every 2-3 years

Patients for the ocular hypertension treatment study (Ch. Introduction II) were selected excluding myopes, labile diabetics, poor compliance. In most of Europe black Africans are a minority.

NOTE:
Assess each patient individually when deciding whether or not to treat.

4.3.1 - SECONDARY OPEN-ANGLE GLAUCOMAS CAUSED BY OPHTHALMOLOGICAL DISEASE

4.3.1.1 - Pseudoexfolation glaucoma

a) Topical medication
b) ALT often achieves a large IOP decrease
c) Filtering procedure

4.3.1.2 - Pigmentary glaucoma

a) Topical medication
   Beware that drugs which dilate the pupil may cause additional pigment liberation and therefore a spike in IOP. Check peripheral retina for tears before using pilocarpine.
b) ALT
   The heavily pigmented trabecular meshwork warrants power lower than usual. The IOP response is highly variable.
c) Filtering procedure
d) Peripheral Nd:YAG laser iridotomy for eliminating reverse pupillary block if present. The potential long-term benefit could be decreased iris rubbing and pigmentary release with a prophylactic role by preventing irreversible trabecular damage.

4.3.1.3 - Lens-induced open-angle glaucoma

Topical anti-inflammatory medication followed by extraction of lens or lens fragments, and vitrectomy if needed

4.3.1.4 - Glaucoma associated with intraocular haemorrhage

a) Topical and systemic IOP lowering medication as needed
b) Paracentesis and wash-out of the anterior chamber
c) Vitrectomy (for vitreous blood)

4.3.1.5 - Uveitic glaucoma

a) Topical and systemic anti-inflammatory therapy
b) Topical and systemic IOP lowering medication as needed
c) Treatment of the underlying disease
d) Glaucoma surgery (consider antimetabolites)

4.3.1.6 - Glaucoma due to intraocular tumor

a) Irradiation, surgical tumor excision, enucleation
b) Topical and systemic IOP lowering medication as needed
c) Cyclodestruction
d) Trabeculectomy not indicated

4.3.1.7 - Glaucoma associated with retinal detachment

a) Topical and systemic IOP lowering medication as needed
b) Surgery for retinal detachment, vitrectomy, cryosurgery, filtration surgery

4.3.1.8 - Open-angle glaucoma due to ocular trauma

a) Anti-inflammatory treatment
b) Topical and systemic IOP lowering medication as needed
c) Long-term follow up with measurement of intraocular pressure since rise in intraocular pressure after trauma may be delayed for years
d) Filtering procedure

4.3.2 - IATROGENIC SECONDARY OPEN-ANGLE GLAUCOMAS

4.3.2.1 - Glaucoma due to corticosteroid treatment

a) Discontinue corticosteroid medication
b) Topical and systemic IOP lowering medication as needed
c) Filtration surgery

4.3.2.2 - Secondary open-angle glaucoma due to ocular surgery and laser

a) Topical and systemic IOP lowering medication as needed
b) Anti-inflammatory treatment
c) Removal silicone oil or the intraocular lens

4.3.3 - SECONDARY OPEN-ANGLE GLAUCOMA CAUSED BY EXTRABULBAR DISEASE

4.3.3.1 - Glaucoma caused by increased episcleral venous pressure

a) Treatment of the underlying disease
b) Topical and systemic IOP lowering medication
c) Surgery according to the specific condition

4.4.1 - PRIMARY ANGLE-CLOSURE (PAC)

Angle-closure with plateau iris mechanism

See FC X
Medical treatment:

Pupillary constriction to pull centripetally the peripheral iris.

In plateau iris configuration, a modest pupillary constriction may prevent further angle-closure

- pilocarpine 1%, aceclidine 2%, carbachol 0.75%
- dapiprazole 0.5%, thymoxamine 0.5%

Surgical treatment:

- Peripheral laser iridoplasty stretches the iris and deepens the chamber angle.
- Iridectomy or Iridotomy may be helpful only when plateau iris is combined with pupillary block mechanism

Angle-closure with posterior aqueous misdirection

See FC X
Medical treatment

- Parasympatholytics (atropine, scopolamine, cyclopentolate) may be useful as a prophylactic or curative regimen.
- Aqueous production suppressants (see above) given orally and/or topically
- Hyperosmotics (Ch. 4.3.1)

Surgical treatment

- A patent iridotomy must be present or, if not present, iridotomy should be performed.
- YAG laser vitreolysis/capsulotomy, especially in aphakia, pseudophakia.
- Anterior vitrectomy, especially in aphakia, pseudophakia.
- In selected cases lens/IOL extraction.

4.4.1.1 - Acute angle-closure with pupillary block mechanism

See FC XI

Iridotomy or iridectomy is the preferred definitive treatment of acute angle-closure glaucoma with a pupillary block component.

Medical treatment only serves to lower IOP, to relieve the symptoms and signs so that laser iridotomy or iridectomy is possible. The main principles of medical therapy aim at

(1) *withdrawal of aqueous from vitreous body and posterior chamber by hyperosmotics,*
(2) *pupillary constriction to free the chamber angle,* and
(3) *reduction of aqueous production,*

ALL THE FOLLOWING THREE STEPS SHOULD BE IMPLEMENTED CONCURRENTLY

- **Reduction of aqueous production**
  - acetazolamide 10 mg/Kg intravenously or orally.
  - topical alpha-2 agonists
  - topical betablockers

Topical CAIs are not potent enough to break pupillary block.

- **Withdrawal of aqueous from vitreous body and posterior chamber**

Hyperosmotics are the most effective agents[5]. The patients must be evaluated for heart or kidney disease because hyperosmotics increase blood volume which increases the load on the heart. Some may alter glucose blood levels and should not be given to diabetics (see FC X).

- Glycerol 1.0 - 1.5 g/Kg orally
- Mannitol 1.0 - 1.5 g/Kg intravenously

- **Pupillary constriction**

  - pilocarpine 1% or 2% or aceclidine 2% twice or three times within 1 hour

Note:
while the sphincter is ischaemic and the pupil non-reactive to light [sphincter paresis], multiple application of parasympathomimetics is not helpful, will not cause pupillary constriction and may cause forward rotation of the ciliary muscle, thereby increasing the pupillary block. Miotics in large doses can cause systemic side effects since they are absorbed transnasally and can cause abdominal cramps. It is now recognised that intensive parasimpathomimetic are no longer indicated to treat this condition. Miotics will constrict the pupil only after IOP has been lowered.

- dapiprazole 0.5% (Glamidolo, Remydrial, RevEyes) or thymoxamine 0.5%. These are alpha-1 blockers that relax the dilator muscle. They do not reduce pupil size when the sphincter-muscle is paretic.

<u>Surgical treatment</u>

- Neodymium YAG laser iridotomy.

Laser iridotomy should be attempted if the cornea is sufficiently clear. Some glaucomatologists prefer surgical iridectomy in all cases of manifest angle-closure glaucoma and use laser iridotomy only as prophylactic treatment of the contralateral eye and in cases of 'occludable angle'. Argon laser iridotomy is rarely performed nowdays.

- Surgical iridectomy

1) Transcorneal approach.

Advantages: no conjunctival scarring
a water-tight self-sealing incision is possible.
Disadvantages: technically more difficult in dilated fixed pupil and flat anterior chamber.

2) Corneoscleral approach.

Advantages: iridectomy can be 'basal'.
Disadvantages: conjunctival wound may lead to scarring compromising the outcome of a filtering procedure which may become necessary at a later stage
insufficient wound closure and aqueous misdirection may occur in rare cases.

General advantages of surgical iridectomy:
it can be performed even when the cornea is cloudy
it allows deepening of the anterior chamber, breaking freshly formed PAS.
General disadvantages of surgical iridectomy:
all the potential risks of any intraocular procedure.

4.4.1.2 - Intermittent Angle-Closure Glaucoma (IACG)

Pupillary constriction, iridotomy, iridoplasty or lens extraction are to be considered according to the main mechanism determining angle occlusion.

4.4.1.3 - Chronic angle-closure glaucoma

Medical treatment rarely effective
If the synechial closure is less than half the circumference, iridectomy/iridotomy may be sufficient. Since complications of iridectomy/iridotomy are uncommon, its use as the initial procedure is justified in practically every case.

Argon laser trabeculoplasty is not indicated as it may increase synechial angle-closure.

If IOP cannot be controlled, a filtering procedure is indicated. These eyes are more frequently prone to develop posterior aqueous misdirection and the necessary precautions must be taken when considering surgery.
Early cataract removal may be considered and could relieve the problem

4.4.3 - THE "OCCLUDABLE" ANGLE; ACR (ANGLE-CLOSURE RISK)

If fellow eye of primary angle-closure, treatment is clearly indicated, starting with laser iridotomy. All other cases must be assessed individually. In general, the risks of laser treatment are to be balanced againts the perceived risk of angle-closure.

4.5 - SECONDARY ANGLE-CLOSURE GLAUCOMAS

4.5.1 - SECONDARY ANGLE-CLOSURE GLAUCOMAS WITH PUPILLARY BLOCK

Several steps may be considered, according to the clinical picture of causative mechanisms.

a) Topical and systemic IOP lowering medication
b) Nd:YAG laser iridotomy
c) Peripheral iridectomy
d) Lens extraction, vitrectomy
e) Discontinuing miotics in miotic-induced pupillary block
f) Pupillary dilation
g) Nd:YAG laser synechiolysis of posterior synechiae

4.5.2 - SECONDARY ANGLE-CLOSURE GLAUCOMAS WITH ANTERIOR "PULLING" MECHANISM WITHOUT PUPILLARY BLOCK

4.5.2.1 - Neovascular glaucoma

a) Topical atropine or equivalent
b) Topical steroid initially
c) Topical and systemic IOP lowering medication as needed
d) Retinal ablation with laser or cryotherapy
e) Cyclodestruction
f) Filtering procedure with antimetabolites
g) Aqueous drainage devices

Miotics are contraindicated

4.5.2.2 - Iridocorneal endothelial syndrome

a) Topical and systemic IOP lowering medications as needed
b) Filtering procedure, with antimetabolite according to risk factors
c) Aqueous drainage device

4.5.2.3 - Posterior polymorphous dystrophy

a) Topical and systemic IOP lowering medication as needed
b) Filtering procedure, with antimetabolite according to risk factors

4.5.2.4 - Peripheral anterior synechiae due to prolonged primary angle-closure glaucoma

a) Topical and systemic IOP lowering medication as needed
b) Filtering procedure

4.5.2.5 - Epithelial and fibrous ingrowth after anterior segment surgery or penetrating trauma

a) Topical and systemic IOP lowering medication as needed
b) Excision, destruction of the immigrated tissue
c) Filtering procedure, with antimetabolite according to risk factors
d) Aqueous drainage device
e) Cyclodestruction

4.5.2.6 - Inflammatory membrane

a) Anti-inflammatory medications and cycloplegics
b) Topical and systemic IOP lowering medication as needed
c) Filtering procedure with antimetabolite
d) Aqueous drainage device
e) Cyclodestruction

4.5.2.7 - Peripheral anterior synechiae after ALT and endothelial membrane covering the trabecular meshwork late after ALT

a) Topical and systemic IOP lowering medication as needed
b) Filtering procedure

4.5.2.8 - Aniridia

a) Topical and systemic IOP lowering medication as needed
b) Trabeculotomy
c) Filtering procedure with antimetabolites
d) Aqueous drainage device
e) Cyclodestruction

4.5.3 - SECONDARY ANGLE-CLOSURE GLAUCOMAS WITH POSTERIOR "PUSHING" MECHANISM WITHOUT PUPILLARY BLOCK

4.5.3.1 - Aqueous misdirection glaucoma

a) Long-term pupillary dilation and cycloplegia
b) Topical and systemic IOP lowering medication as needed
c) Laser or surgical dissection of the anterior hyaloid face or lens capsule and/or iridotomy
d) Vitrectomy with dissection of the anterior hyaloid face
Miotics are contraindicated

4.5.3.2 - Iris and ciliary body cysts, intraocular tumors

a) Topical and systemic IOP lowering medication as needed
b) Cyst destruction with laser or surgical excision
c) Tumor irradiation
d) Filtering surgery
e) Cyclodestruction

4.5.3.3 - Silicon oil or gas implanted in the vitreous cavity

a) Topical/systemic IOP lowering medications as needed
b) Silicon oil or gas aspiration
c) Filtering surgery
d) Drainage device
e) Cyclodestruction

4.5.3.4 - Uveal effusion due to

1. inflammation (scleritis, uveitis, HIV infection)
2. increased choroidal venous pressure (nanophthalmos, scleral buckling, panretinal photocoagulation, central retinal vein occlusion, artero-venous communication)
3. tumor

a) Anti-inflammatory medication (for 1)
b) Topical and systemic IOP lowering medication as needed (for 1, 2 and 3)
c) Relaxation of scleral buckling; vitrectomy, sclerectomy in nanophthalmus (for 2)
d) Tumor excision or irradiation (for 3)
e) Cyclodestruction (for 1, 2 and 3)

4.5.3.5 - Retinopathy of prematurity (stage V)

a) Topical and systemic IOP lowering medications
b) Cyclodestruction
c) Filtering procedure with or without antimetabolite
d) Drainage devices

4.5.3.6 - Congenital anomalies that can be associated with secondary glaucoma

Treatment to be adapted to the primary anomaly, the mechanism of IOP elevation and the quality of life of the patient

References

For references, see corresponding topics in Ch. 2 and Ch. 3.

NOTES

NOTES

NOTES

NOTES

NOTES